Simple Keto Instant Pot

Cookbook 2018

Quick, Easy and Delicious Low Carb High Fat Ketogenic Diet
Recipes to Lose Weight Fast, Prevent Disease, and Be Longevity

By Dr. Mark Pitre

INTRODUCTION

Do you want to have a bible of Ketogenic Diet just in one book?
Do you want to have many mouth-watering and easy-to-make instant pot recipes?
Do you want to combine both to serve you and upgrade your living?

If yes of any questions above, then this book is definitely for you! This book *written by **Dr. Mark Pitre*** is the most comprehensive and actionable guide on the ketogenic diet that discusses not only the complete guidelines (foods to eat and avoid, tips for success, and so on) but also provides many simple delicious and easy-to-prepare recipes that you can prepare at home.

Ketogenic diet nowadays is the most popular diet around the world! Originally designed for patients with epilepsy, the ketogenic diet has also been discovered to be an effective weight loss tool, helping people shed unwanted pounds and at the same time, promoting overall health.

In this book, we shall discuss everything that you need to know about Ketogenic Diet. ***No matter if you are a beginner or the ones who have already dived into Keto Diet for a period of time, this book must be your first choice!*** This book will tell you every point in detail and in a scientific way, not only tell you the truth, but also tell you the reasons. Just keep on reading, you will like it and cherish it!

Since it can be quite challenging getting started on any diet program, we have provided recipes that are not only easy to cook, but also are conveniently prepared using the Instant Pot. In the latter part of the book, you will find tips and guidelines that will help you use the Instant Pot successfully.

Good luck on your journey to a healthier you!

Table of Contents

CHAPTER 1 – BASIC INFORMATION

WHAT IS THE KETOGENIC DIET?

The ketogenic diet comes in various names—low carb diet, low carb high fat diet, keto diet, and so on.

Basically, it is based on the principle of encouraging the body to produce ketones as energy source.

Here's how it works:

When people eat foods that are rich in carbohydrates, the body produces **glucose** and **insulin**.

Glucose can easily be converted into energy, which is why the body prefers it as energy source.

Insulin, meanwhile, is produced so that the body can use it to process the glucose.

If the body uses glucose as energy source, fats take a backseat. They are not utilized, and are instead stored in the tissues. The more fats stored, the more a person gains weight.

If you reduce the intake of carbohydrates, the body goes through a process of **ketosis**. During this process, the body breaks down the fats from the food eaten and from those that are stored in the tissues. As a result, the body produces ketones, and this is what it uses for energy.

WHO SHOULD FOLLOW THE KETOGENIC DIET?

The ketogenic is ideal for most people who want to lose weight, prevent ailments, and promote overall health.

As mentioned earlier, it is designed for people who suffer from epilepsy. Its efficacy as treatment aid has been proven in scientific research (https://www.ncbi.nlm.nih.gov/pmc/articles/PMC2902940/).

Athletes who want to power up fat metabolism are also encouraged to adopt this diet program.

It's important to know however that this diet is not for everyone.

It is not recommended for people who have been diagnosed with any kidney disease, liver disease or pancreatic disease. Although this has been used by diabetic patients, anyone who has any blood sugar issues should first consult a doctor before using this diet.

Moreover, pregnant and nursing women are not advised to follow the keto diet.

WHAT DOES KETOSIS MEAN?

Ketosis is a metabolic process that a body undergoes when it does not receive enough carbohydrates to use for energy. In order to keep working, the body looks for alternative source of energy so it turns to the fat stored in your tissues or those obtained from foods that you consume.

As mentioned earlier, this process produces organic compounds called **ketones**, which the body converts into energy. This is the main principle by which the ketogenic diet works—by prompting the body to go into ketosis through a low carb diet, it burns fat instead of carbs, helping you lose weight along the way.

HOW TO IDENTIFY IF YOU ARE IN KETOSIS OR NOT

There are two ways to determine if you have reached the state of ketosis:
- Measure the ketones inside your body
- Look for signs and symptoms of ketosis

Ways to Measure Ketones

To measure ketone level, you can use the following tools:
- **Urine sticks** – A urine stick is a cheap device that you can use to measure the number of ketones in your body. However, the accuracy rate is quite low.
- **Breath ketone meter** – This is used to measure the ketones in your breath. It is more expensive than the urine stick but more accurate.
- **Blood ketone meter** – This is the most expensive and most accurate tool that you can use to measure ketone level in the body.

Signs and Symptoms of Ketosis

Watch out for these signs and symptoms so you will know if you have reached the state of ketosis or not.
- **More frequent urination** – The keto diet is a natural diuretic.
- **Dry mouth** – This is usually accompanied by increased thirst.
- **Bad breath** – Bad breath is caused by the acetone by product from the ketones that are partially excreted through the breath.
- **Increased energy levels** – Once your body has adjusted to the diet, you will feel more energetic.

- **Reduced hunger** – The keto diet has also been proven to reduce hunger pangs and suppress cravings especially for sweets.

HOW CAN I GET INTO KETOSIS?

Reaching the state of ketosis is actually very simple. The steps are outlined below:
- **Reduce intake of carbohydrates** – To get optimal results, one needs to reduce intake not only of net carbs but also of total carbs. It's ideal to limit intake to 20 grams net carbs and 35 grams total carbs per day.
- **Limit protein consumption** – Most people focus only on the carb intake, not realizing that protein should also be reduced. It's important to keep in mind that excessive protein can hamper the process of ketosis. It's best to keep your protein intake to 0.6 grams and 0.8 grams per pound of lean body mass. Use a keto calculator (https://www.ruled.me/keto-calculator)to help you determine your ideal protein intake.
- **Don't reduce fat intake** – Fat will be the main source of energy for your body while you're on the ketogenic diet so there's no need to limit intake. However, it'd be a good idea to rely more on healthy fats (http://www.health.com/health/gallery/0,,20477647,00.html).
- **Keep yourself hydrated** – As mentioned earlier, dry mouth and increased thirst are some of the symptoms of ketosis. This is why, you need to drink eight to 10 glasses of water or more a day. This will help regulate the essential bodily processes as well as reduce hunger pangs.
- **Limit snacking** – Snacking slows down weight loss and spikes up the insulin levels.
- **Get regular exercise** – It's not wise to take on any weight loss diet without exercise. Aim for at least 30 minutes of moderate aerobic exercise a day.

Basically, you need to maintain this percentage of macronutrients:
- **Fats** – 60 to 80 percent of daily calories
- **Protein** – 20 to 25 percent of daily calories
- **Carbohydrates** – 5 to 10 percent of daily calories

WHAT ARE KETONES?

Also called **ketone bodies**, ketones refer to the by-products of the body after it metabolizes fat to be used for energy.
There are three types of ketones:
- Acetoacetate (AcAc)

- Beta-hydroxybutyric acid (BHB)
- Acetone

Acetoacetate and beta-hydroxybutyrate transport energy from the liver to other parts of the body. Meanwhile, acetone is a by-product that is excreted through urine or breath.

REQUIRED QUANTITY OF CARB INTAKE

It's important to know that people have different carb limits. Generally, it is advised to stay below 35 grams of total carbs and 25 grams of net carbs.

You can determine net carbs by subtracting fiber grams from the total carbs. Staying within this limit helps you achieve ketosis and maintain this metabolic state. But as said earlier, it's also important not to consume excessive amounts of protein.

KETO DIET VS. ATKINS DIET

The Atkins Diet became popular in the early 2000s as a diet program promoting weight loss and better health. It was introduced by Dr. Robert Coleman Atkins, after discovering in 1963 that carbohydrate reduction resulted in weight loss.

This diet has undergone many changes but currently, there are two main types:

- **Atkins 20** – This is designed for people who intend to lose more than 40 pounds of weight.
- **Atkins 40** – This is a less-restrictive type for those who intend to lose less than 40 pounds of weight.

Compared to the Atkins Diet, the ketogenic diet appears to have more benefits.

For one, keto is more a lifestyle while Atkins is a short-term weight loss program. With the latter, there's less chance of maintaining long-term results.

With the Atkins Diet, carbs are re-introduced into the diet after the initial phase. In the phases following the initial stage, people are prompted to consume up to 100 grams of carbs a day.

This leads to the person gaining back the weight that he initially lost. This scenario does not happen with ketogenic dieters as long as they continue following the program.

During the initial phase, the two diet programs appear to be similar. But most people who have tried both diet programs can attest that keto is what you should go for if you want long-lasting results.

LOW CARB DIET VS. KETO DIET

Keto is often called the low carb diet, but it's important to realize that a low carb diet is actually different.

While both types of diet programs limit carb intake, take note that the keto diet also regulates protein consumption. Lowering intake of carbohydrates is futile if you keep consuming too much protein.

Excessive protein is known to hamper the process of ketosis. It is for this reason that many people find the keto diet more effective than any other low carb diet program.

CHAPTER 2: ADVANTAGES OF KETOGENIC DIET

One of the reasons the keto diet has become popular all over the world is not only because it is effective as a weight loss program, but also because it has many other benefits for the health.

Below, you will understand how the keto diet helps you shed unwanted pounds, and at the same time, keep you in top shape.

BALANCING YOUR BLOOD SUGAR LEVELS

A high level of blood sugar is not good for you. It causes unpleasant side effects such as fatigue, headache, difficulty in concentrating, and blurry vision, among others.

Not only that, it also shoots up the risk of type 2 diabetes. The CDC (https://www.cdc.gov/media/releases/2014/p0610-diabetes-report.html) reports that in the United States alone, there are now over 29 million people who suffer from this condition. What's the cause? Experts agree that type 2 diabetes can be a result of unhealthy diet and lifestyle. Processed food products such as cakes, candies and pastries, as well as naturally starchy foods like potatoes and rice can increase blood sugar levels.

You'll know that you have high blood sugar levels if you experience increased thirst, headaches, frequent urination, weakness, and unexplained weight loss. Blood sugar that is more than 180 mg/dL is considered high.

If this happens frequently, it can lead to the following:

- Blood floor reduction
- Increased risk of stroke, heart attack and type 2 diabetes
- Nerve damage
- Blindness
- Kidney failure

The good news is you can prevent type 2 diabetes along with other chronic ailments, and control blood sugar levels with the help of the ketogenic diet.

The keto diet has been found to be more effective than low-calorie diets in reducing the risk of these ailments.

In a study (https://www.ncbi.nlm.nih.gov/pmc/articles/PMC1325029/) published in the *Nutrition & Metabolism Journal*, it was found that the keto diet can successfully improve high blood sugar levels, and even reduce the intake of medications among patients diagnosed with type 2 diabetes.

A total of 28 overweight patients with diabetes underwent a 16-week study in which they were asked to undergo a diet that reduced daily carb intake to less than 20 grams.

Results showed that the body mass index (BMI) for most of the participants reduced significantly. The blood sugar level also decreased, and a few of the patients were able to discontinue or reduce the use of medications.

Despite these findings, it is important to remember that one should consult a doctor first before taking on the keto diet as treatment aid for diabetes.

MANAGING YOUR BLOOD PRESSURE LEVELS

Like blood sugar levels, blood pressure levels should also be controlled.

Blood pressure refers to the amount of pressure exerts by the blood on the blood vessel walls. This is determined through two numbers:

- **Systolic pressure** – This is the top number which is the amount of the pressure in the arteries during heart contraction.
- **Diastolic pressure** – This indicates the pressure in the arteries during the beating of the heart.

Both numbers are express in millimetres of mercury (mm Hg).

The standard or healthy blood pressure level is 120/80 mm Hg. If a person has 121/81 mm Hg to 139/90 mm Hg blood pressure level, he/she will typically be diagnosed with pre-hypertension.

If not given immediate attention, this can lead to hypertension. Hypertension is a condition characterized by blood pressure levels above 140/90 mm Hg. This can lead to several complications such as kidney failure, stroke, heart attack, heart failure, and even death.

According to the Blood Pressure UK (http://www.bloodpressureuk.org/mediacentre/FAQs), one in three adults has high blood pressure. This is quite alarming, and should be given sufficient attention.

Managing blood pressure levels is possible with the right diet and regular exercise. It's also important to regularly undergo blood pressure screening.

Research has shown that the keto diet can help maintain proper levels of blood pressure.

A study (https://www.ncbi.nlm.nih.gov/pmc/articles/PMC4666896/) conducted by a team of scientists from Italy reported that the keto diet can improve various cardiovascular risk factors including high blood pressure. Researchers recommend further randomized trials to confirm their findings.

For most people, this can be quite surprising since high fat diets have always been associated with high blood pressure.

A 2015 study (http://europepmc.org/abstract/med/26602244) counters this with evidence showing that a low fat, high carb diet can actually increase blood pressure levels.

If you have been diagnosed with prehypertension or hypertension, check with your doctor first before undergoing the keto diet.

MAINTAINING PROPER CHOLESTEROL LEVELS

One of the most popular misconceptions about the keto diet is that because it's high in fat, it automatically shoots up cholesterol levels.

But research has proven otherwise. Recent studies show that a low carb diet can in fact lower cholesterol levels and reduce the risk of heart disease.

Before we get to that, it's important to first understand the functions of cholesterol and fat in the body.

Also called lipids, fats are molecules known to repel water. It is present in the bloodstream in two forms:

- **Triglycerides** – This refers to a fatty acid that stores energy, and can be metabolized to be used as fuel. An increase in the triglycerides can lead to the onset of heart disease and diabetes.
- **Cholesterol** – This refers to the waxy substance that has many roles in the body such as producing hormones, helping absorb vitamins, strengthens the cell membranes and so on. This substance is produced by the body through the liver. It can also be derived from foods such as red meat, dairy and poultry.

Cholesterol can be further broken down into five forms:

- Chylomicrons
- Very-low-density lipoproteins (VLDL)
- Intermediate-density lipoproteins (IDL)
- Low-density lipoproteins (LDL)
- High-density lipoproteins (HDL)

In this section, we are going to focus more on the HDL and LDL cholesterol.

HDL cholesterol is often called the "good cholesterol". Its primary role is to transport cholesterol throughout the body, and to collect those that not utilized by the cells so that it can either be recycled or removed in the liver.

It has been dubbed as the good cholesterol because it prevents cholesterol from building up and clogging the arteries. Having high HDL levels is actually good for the health.

The ideal range for HDL is 40 to 60 mg/dl for men, and 50 to 60 mg/dl for women.

LDL cholesterol, on the other hand, is referred to as the "bad cholesterol". But it's more complicated than most people realize. Yes, the LDL also helps in the transportation of the cholesterol in the body.

The problem is, it is more susceptible to oxidation by harmful substances called **free radicals**. Aside from that, the LDL can also attach to the arterial walls and hamper proper functioning of the heart.

This is why an increase in LDL cholesterol levels can be quite alarming as this means that you will be at an increased risk of heart disease.

It's ideal to maintain LDL levels at below 100 mg/dL. Some people can have LDL levels of up to 129 mg/dL without experiencing any problem. However, those who have health issues or are at risk of heart disease should make an effort to maintain proper LDL cholesterol level. In 2004, researchers from Kuwait (https://www.ncbi.nlm.nih.gov/pmc/articles/PMC2716748/)evaluated the effects of a 24-week ketogenic diet among obese patients.

A total of 83 obese patients with BMI greater than 35 kg/m2 and who suffer from high cholesterol levels participated in this study. Aside from the body weight, the participants' HDL, LDL and triglyceride levels were also measured.

After the study, it was found that the BMI of the participants decreased significantly. It was also noted in the findings that the HDL cholesterol levels increased while the LDL cholesterol and triglyceride levels were reduced. Researchers confirmed that the keto diet has positive effects on cholesterol levels.

HELPING IN WEIGHT LOSS

For most people, losing weight is all about looking better, and feeling more confident. But what many take for granted is how maintaining the right weight can help avert many types of illnesses.

Obesity has been linked to numerous conditions including heart disease, stroke, diabetes, certain types of cancer, gallbladder disease, osteoarthritis, gout, and breathing problems. Alarmingly, obesity has become a major problem in many parts of the world. The WHO (http://www.who.int/news-room/fact-sheets/detail/obesity-and-overweight)reports that obesity has increased in trifold since 1975, and that over 1.9 billion people are overweight.

Adopting a healthy diet is a step towards healthy weight loss. Many studies have provided evidence that the keto diet is effective in helping people lose weight.

Although primarily designed as treatment for epilepsy, the keto diet's claim to fame in the modern society is its ability to shed unwanted pounds. More and more people are using this diet program as a weight loss tool, and have found success in doing so.

A meta-analysis (https://www.ncbi.nlm.nih.gov/pubmed/23651522/)of several randomized controlled trials showed that the keto diet is highly effective in reducing weight and BMI. Researchers noted that those who use the low carbohydrate diet lost significantly more weight than those who adopted the low-fat diet, indicating that very low carb keto diet can be an "alternative tool against obesity".

REGULATING YOUR APPETITE

A benefit related to weight loss is the keto diet's ability to regulate the appetite.

As we all know, cravings are some of the major hindrances in a dieter's weight loss journey. It becomes a lot more difficult to lose weight if you are constantly craving for unhealthy snacks and treats.

According to Mind Body Green (https://www.mindbodygreen.com/articles/a-doctor-on-why-ketosis-helps-you-lose-weight), ketosis is a "**great appetite suppressant**". Anyone following a standard western diet that's high in carbohydrates is prone to experience "blood sugar swings" that cause hunger pangs. Sometimes, one will start to crave for food only one to two hours after finishing meal.

But once you're in the process of ketosis, the body will start to burn fat for energy, which in turn stabilizes the blood sugar levels. Fat will be metabolized in the liver. As a result, hunger pangs will be reduced significantly.

Moreover, ketosis also affects the levels of **ghrelin**, which is the hunger hormone that makes you want to eat more. When you're in a keto diet, the ghrelin hormone drops, and you will no longer experience frequent cravings.

This is not a baseless claim. In fact, it was noted in a 2014 study (https://www.ncbi.nlm.nih.gov/pmc/articles/PMC3945587/) published in the *International Journal of Environmental Research and Public Health* that the keto diet reduces appetite through the satiety effect of protein intake and effect on hunger hormones. It is also believed that the ketone bodies also have "appetite suppressant action".

GETTING RID OF VISCERAL FAT

More popularly known as belly fat, **visceral fat** is not only unsightly but also dangerous. This type of deep gel-like fat that covers major organs such as the kidneys, liver and pancreas can increase the risk of the following diseases:

- Cancer
- Heart disease
- Stroke
- Diabetes
- Dementia
- Depression
- Arthritis
- Sexual dysfunction

Aside from increasing the risk of these conditions, the excess fat can also disrupt the normal functioning of the hormones, and at the same time, promote the production of pro-inflammatory chemicals known as **cytokines**.

Most people who have belly fat will probably agree that it can be very difficult to get rid of.

The good news is, you can finally say goodbye to stubborn belly fat with the help of the keto diet.

But before we get to that, let's first understand why it's challenging to remove belly fat.

To understand what makes belly fat so difficult to burn, let's dive into the biology.

Burning fat has two stages:

- **Lipolysis** – This refers to the process in which the fat cells release the molecules of stored fat into the bloodstream.
- **Oxidation** – In the process of oxidation, cells burn the stored fat.

The process of lipolysis is stimulated by **catecholamines**, which may be impeded by alpha receptors and triggered by beta receptors.

Visceral fat contains fat cells that have more alpha receptors, which explains why it is more difficult than other types of fat to burn.

When one undergoes a ketogenic diet, the body has no choice but to burn fat for energy, even the stubborn ones such as the fat in the belly area. It's for this reason that those who struggle with visceral fat have found great success in the keto diet.

HELPING WITH METABOLIC SYNDROME

Metabolic syndrome is not just one condition. It is actually a cluster of several conditions including high blood pressure, high blood sugar, high cholesterol and excess visceral fat, all occurring at the same time, shooting up the risk for diabetes, stroke and heart disease.

The exact cause is unknown. However, experts agree that it is triggered by obesity and sedentary lifestyle. It can also be associated with insulin resistance.

If you are at risk of metabolic syndrome or have been diagnosed with this condition, the keto diet can certainly help.

In a 2017 study (https://static1.squarespace.com/static/59ae01e849fc2b19c93fbb46/t/5a028ceeec212d79d86caf4e/1510116592216/Diabetes+%26+Metabolic+Syndrome-+Clinical+Research+%26+Reviews.pdf)conducted by American researchers, it was reported that the keto diet may reverse the process that triggers that onset of metabolic syndrome.

A group of 30 patients diagnosed with metabolic syndrome participated in this experiment. The first group followed a keto diet with no exercise. The second group used the standard American diet with no exercise. The third group was required to undergo the standard American diet with 30 minutes of daily exercise for five days.

After 10 weeks, findings revealed that the first group had significant reduction in BMI, body fat percentage and weight. They also had lower levels of A1C (https://medlineplus.gov/a1c.html)(a measure of average blood glucose).

It was concluded that the keto diet was effective than the standard American diet even when combined with exercise in reducing the risk of metabolic syndrome.

HELPING WITH COGNITIVE DISORDERS

Cognitive disorders remain a major issue in many countries around the world. The WHO (http://www.who.int/bulletin/volumes/91/10/13-118422/en/)estimates that there are currently about 35 million people who suffer from dementia worldwide. The rate is expected to double in 20 years.

Also called neurocognitive disorders, cognitive disorders refer to a classification of mental health problems that disrupt cognitive skills and abilities including memory, learning, problem solving and perception, among others.

Some of the most common cognitive disorders are dementia, autism and Down syndrome. Dyslexia and attention deficit disorder (ADD) are also considered as cognitive conditions but are less severe.

Although the keto diet cannot treat or reverse Down Syndrome and other cognitive conditions, it has been found to be effective in enhancing memory among elderly people with mild cognitive impairment.

A team of American researchers (https://www.ncbi.nlm.nih.gov/pmc/articles/PMC3116949/)divided a group of 23 elderly adults with mild cognitive impairment into two groups. The first group followed a high carbohydrate diet while the second group was made to take a low carbohydrate diet.

After six weeks, the researchers noted significant improvement in memory performance among those who followed the low carbohydrate diet.

This positive effect could be attributed to the ability of ketosis to reduce inflammation as well as improve energy metabolism, both of which can lead to better cognitive function.

IMPROVING MENTAL HEALTH

Not surprisingly, the keto diet appears to have a positive effect not only on cognition but on general mental health.

According to its proponents, the keto diet has numerous benefits for the brain, including boosting the mood, enhancing brain function, neutralizing free radical damage, and promoting the production of "feel good" neurotransmitters.

While in ketosis, the brain produces more of the neurotransmitter called **GABA**. Studies have shown that many anxiety related disorders stem from reduced GABA activity in the brain. Experts also agree that increased GABA levels can help reduce stress and anxiety and at the same time, improve mental focus.

Not only that, keto dieters are also found to be at less risk of depression. The ketogenic diet's antidepressive effects were confirmed in a 2004 study (https://www.ncbi.nlm.nih.gov/pubmed/15601609)featured in the *Biological Psychiatry Journal*.

It is also interesting to note that the ketones produced during ketosis can power up the brain more effectively than glucose, as reported in a 2005 study (http://onlinelibrary.wiley.com/doi/10.1002/bmb.2005.49403304246/full).

CHAPTER 3: RISKS AND SYMPTOMS WHEN IN KETO DIET

While it's true that the keto diet has many scientifically proven benefits, it's not without side effects and risks. If you are going to follow this diet, it's very important to know all about these so you can be prepared, and you will know what exactly you have to do.

KETOGENIC FLU

One of the most common complaints among keto dieters is the **keto flu.**
Also called the "carb flu", the keto flu refers to the withdrawal process that the body undergoes after transitioning from a high carb to a low carb diet. It signals that the body is adjusting from using sugar as energy to burning fat for fuel.
According to some keto dieters, this condition is similar to withdrawal from addictive substances, which is not a surprise since sugar has been dubbed as the "cocaine of the food world".
The following are some of the common symptoms of the keto flu:

- Cravings
- Dizziness and lightheadedness
- Brain fog
- Inability to focus
- Nausea
- Muscle camping
- Confusion
- Irritability
- Stomach ache
- Insomnia

For most people, these symptoms last for about a week and can go away without any intervention. But if the keto flu takes longer than two to three weeks, it can be a sign that the body is not adjusting well.
To manage your keto flu symptoms, here are some tips to follow:

- **Replenish your supply of electrolytes** – Drink electrolyte beverages or take electrolyte supplements. Make sure that your electrolyte beverage or supplement does not contain sugar and artificial sweeteners. You can also make your own by mixing one cup water, one teaspoon sea salt and one teaspoon lemon juice.
- **Keep yourself hydrated** – Aside from electrolytes, you also need to make sure that you have enough fluids in your body. If not, you will feel tired, sluggish and will probably suffer from episodes of headaches. Drink eight to 10 glasses of water each day, or even more if you're active.
- **Use bone broth as remedy** – Bone broth is a good remedy for keto flu. Not only does it provide the electrolytes you need (potassium and sodium), it also keeps your body hydrated. Of course, homemade bone broth is the preferred for treating the keto flu.

- **Consume more fat** – Yes, you heard it right. Instead of slowing down on fat intake, you can eat more to help the body adjust more quickly. But remember to load up on healthy fats only such as avocado, olive oil, nuts and seeds and so on.
- **Get moving** – Although you're feeling weak and tired, and would probably want to stay in bed the whole day, the best way to relieve the keto flu symptoms is to get moving. There's no need to engage in strenuous exercises. A gentle walk in the park will do. This will relieve muscle cramping and pain, and at the same time, boost the mood and make you feel better.
- **Get good quality sleep** – Some people complain that the keto flu makes it difficult for them to fall or stay asleep. One thing that you can do is to soak in a warm salt bath. This will effectively relax the muscles and soothe your senses. That's not all, it will also boost the electrolyte absorption. Best to use for this purpose is magnesium salts. It's also a good idea to refrain from using gadgets an hour or two before sleeping. The blue light emitted by smart phones and other tech gadgets disrupt the body's circadian rhythm, making it difficult for a person to fall asleep.

BAD BREATH

Bad breath is a common side effect not only of the keto diet but also of other low carb diets. This is caused by the ketones that in turn produce acetone that's released through the breath. Experts assure that this is not a hygiene issue. Unfortunately, it cannot be resolved with brushing or flossing.

So what can you do instead? Drinking more water helps. It keeps the mouth moist, preventing bacteria from reproducing. It also helps the organs function more effectively, burning fat more easily.

HEADACHES

During the first week of the keto diet, most people suffer from mild to moderate episodes of headaches.

There are three possible causes:
- Dehydration
- Sugar or carbohydrate withdrawal
- Electrolyte imbalance

Some people experience headaches for only one day, while for others the problem can go on for over a week. To resolve this symptom, it's best to keep yourself hydrated with enough water. It also helps to increase consumption of sodium by drinking bone broth.

Headaches can also be averted with the help of supplements. Some of the recommended supplements include:

- L-carnitine
- Co-Enzyme Q10
- Omega-3 fatty acids

Moreover, a few experts recommend avoiding protein during the first phase of the keto diet, limiting intake to 25 percent of overall calorie intake.

LEG CRAMPS

Cramps especially in the legs are a typical occurrence among those who are just starting out on the keto diet. Leg cramps usually take place in the morning or in the evening. It indicates deficiency in minerals, particularly in magnesium.

Drinking plenty of fluids and taking magnesium supplements can help.

TEMPORARY FATIGUE

It's also normal to experience fatigue during the start of the keto diet. When the body is transitioning from one diet to another, it typically undergoes major processes that would make you feel tired and sluggish.

The best way to fight fatigue is with exercise. Yes, you would probably want to get a lot of rest. And that's good too. However, if you want your energy back, you should get moving. A 30-minute mild to moderate intensity aerobic exercise daily is recommended to combat fatigue.

DIFFICULTY SLEEPING

Some people also find it difficult to sleep while on a keto diet. This can be due to the other symptoms such as the keto flu, headaches, or cramping.

As mentioned earlier, soaking in a salt bath can help induce good quality sleep. It's also a must to turn off tech gadgets an hour or two before going to bed.

CONSTIPATION

Constipation is most commonly caused by dehydration. The most effective solution? To increase intake of water, that is. It's also a smart move to take in more fiber from non-starchy vegetables as this helps the bowel to move more efficiently. If this doesn't work to relieve your constipation, try taking in a probiotic or using psyllium husk powder.

CHAPTER 4: WHY YOU'RE NOT PRODUCING ENOUGH KETONES

Achieving ketosis is the primary step in the journey towards the ketogenic diet success. However, not everyone is able to reach this state as immediately as they expect. For some, it seems like no matter what they do, the diet program does not seem to work.

There are some cases in which the body does not produce enough ketones to reach the state of ketosis.

And there are many possible reasons for this. Enumerated below are the reasons deemed by experts as hindrances to ketosis success.

REASON # 1 – EXCESSIVE CONSUMPTION OF PROTEIN

So you've reduced your carb intake and increased consumption of healthy fats. How come the diet is still not working? It's possible that you are consuming too much protein.

When you're on a ketogenic diet, you only need enough amount of protein to help the muscles recover. Take note that if you consume too much of this nutrient, it will prevent the body from achieving the state of ketosis. This is due to **gluconeogenesis**.

Gluconeogenesis refers to a metabolic process in which protein that you consume is converted into glycogen. What happens is that the body remains dependent on glucose as source of energy.

Therefore, it will not use fat as fuel, defeating the primary purpose of ketosis. It's imperative that you consume just the right amount of protein so as not to hamper the process of ketosis from taking place.

REASON # 2 – CONSUMPTION OF HIDDEN CARBOHYDRATES

As much as possible you've tried to stay away from foods with high carbs namely grains, bread, pasta, and so on. In fact, you've done a great job sticking to the foods that are on the "foods to eat" list.

But even so, you're still not getting the results that you're hoping for. The problem? Hidden carbohydrates.

Be aware that there are certain foods like nuts, dairy and some types of vegetables that are in fact keto-approved that contain more carbs than you think.

It's best to consume dairy and nuts in moderation. And if you're going to prepare dishes that contain cruciferous vegetables such as broccoli, cabbage or cauliflower, limit the amount that you'll include.

REASON # 3 – EATING TOO MUCH FOOD

Some people make the mistake of thinking that just because the keto diet is a high fat diet, there's no limit to the amount of fat that they can consume.
But you'd have to remember, if you eat a lot of fat, you're going to end up taking in a lot of calories. As you know, fats have twice more calories than proteins or carbs. This makes it imperative for you to be mindful of your fat intake so you know how many calories you are consuming.
It helps to use a keto macro calculator(https://www.perfectketo.com/keto-macro-calculator/)to determine how many calories you need to take in based on your age, body fat, weight, height, physical activity and weight loss goals.

REASON # 4 – NOT EATING ENOUGH FOOD

Surprisingly, not eating enough food can also have the same effect on your keto diet.
If you're taking in less than the right amount of calories, the body will go into starvation mode and slow down the metabolism to enable you to have energy left to use throughout the day.
This is why, you need to ensure that you're taking in proper number of calories, fat and other nutrients.

REASON # 5 – TOO MUCH EXERCISE

It's true what they say that too much of a good thing can be bad. This is also true with exercise.
Yes, exercise is essential not only to weight loss but to overall health and fitness. However, if you're over exercising, you will end up eating more than you should to replace the burned calories and to keep your energy levels up.
Not only that, over exercising can also increase the risk of internal inflammation and oxidative stress.
Aim for a minimum of 30 minutes of aerobic exercise per day. You can go for as long as one to two hours. But do not spend the whole day jogging or running on the treadmill.

REASON # 6 - STRESS

Stress is a part of most people's daily lives. While it's good to experience stress from time to time as it heightens alertness and helps a person come up with quick actions, chronic stress is bad for the health.

It can also hamper the process of ketosis, preventing weight loss. That's because when one is stressed out, the body releases the hormone cortisol, which is also the one in charge for storing fat in the abdominal area.

If you're on a ketogenic diet but you find yourself constantly stressed out, you need to take a break and make use of stress-reduction techniques to achieve the goals that you want.

Listening to soothing music, taking a warm bath, reading a book or catching up with friends are some of the effective ways to de-stress. You should also try breathing exercises, yoga, meditation and massage therapy, which have worked wonders for people who suffer from chronic stress.

REASON # 7 – LACK OF SLEEP

Another factor that can prevent the body from reaching the state of ketosis is lack of sleep. Sleep deprivation has always been known to be a factor that prevents weight loss.

Here's what happens: if you don't get enough sleep, the circadian rhythms are disrupted, affecting the proper functioning of the body's internal organs. As a result, the body will not burn the calories the way it should.

Sleep also plays an important role in the proper balance of hormones. **Ghrelin**, the hormone that signals hunger, increases due to lack of sleep. This means that you will have more cravings if you're not getting enough eyeshut at night.

REASON # 8 – LEPTIN RESISTANCE

Leptin is a hormone that signals the brain that you're full after eating. It is in charge of regulating the number of calories you take in, the amount of fat stored in the body, and how much of these are burned. This hormone is produced by the fat cells inside the body.

If you suffer from **leptin resistance**, which means that even though the body produces enough of this hormone, the brain does not receive its messages, this can have a negative effect on your ketogenic diet.

Leptin resistance can be caused by a number of factors, the most common of which include lack of sleep, unhealthy diet, stress, over eating, and slow metabolism. You need to do something about leptin resistance to be able to get to your goals more quickly.

REASON # 9 – FOOD SENSITIVITY

Some people have sensitivities to certain types of food without even knowing it.
For example, you might be sensitive to dairy, and this might be causing an imbalance in your digestive tract without you being aware of it. This can lead to inflammation, which in turn contributes to weight gain as well as increases the risk of a number of diseases.
If you suspect that you have any food sensitivity, monitor your reaction to certain foods and determine which ones you should avoid or limit intake of.

CHAPTER 5: SHOPPING GUIDE OF KETOGENIC DIET

When you're on the ketogenic diet (or any diet program), grocery shopping can be a lot more challenging.

Each time you'd pick a product, you'd have to think twice, thrice or many times if you can actually buy and consume that product, or if it will ruin your diet program.

To make things easier for you, we've rounded up a list of foods that you can eat and foods that are not allowed.

FOODS YOU CAN EAT

If you're wondering which specific types of food are allowed in this diet program, here's a list of what you should eat more often.

Fats and Oils

As mentioned in the previous chapters, you'll be getting most of your caloric intake from fats. But take note that you can't just devour whatever fat you get your hands on. You need to be picky, and include in your diet those that will not harm your health.

Basically, there are three types of fat allowed in the ketogenic diet:

- **Saturated fat** – Coconut oil, lard, ghee and butter
- **Monounsaturated fat** – Olive oil, macadamia nut oil, avocado oil
- **Polyunsaturated fat** – Fatty fish (wild salmon, trout, tuna), meat protein, non-hydrogenated animal fat

Other good sources of healthy fat:

- Tallow
- Egg yolk
- Brazil nuts
- Mayonnaise
- Cocoa butter
- Coconut butter
- Avocado
- MCT oil

When using vegetable oils such as olive oil or soybean oil, always go for the cold-pressed options. If you are going to cook in high heat, it's better to use oils with higher smoke points such as ghee and coconut oil.

Protein

Protein is also a vital part of the ketogenic diet. Consuming too little or too much can wreak havoc to your diet program.

When looking for protein sources, here are some key points to keep in mind:

- Go for grass-fed and pasture-raised meat
- Choose darker meat than white meat
- Be wary of hidden sugars and additives in sausages and cured meat
- Select fattier cuts of meat such as rib eye

Preferred protein sources:

- **Fish** – Cod, flounder, salmon, tuna, catfish, halibut, mahi-mahi, mackerel, snapper
- **Seafood** – Oysters, crabs, mussels, clams, lobster, scallops, squid
- **Eggs** – Free-range chicken, duck or turkey eggs
- **Beef** – Steak, stew met, ground beef, roasts
- **Pork** – Pork chops, pork tenderloin, pork loin
- **Poultry** – Chicken, quail, duck, wild game
- **Offal/organ** – Animal liver, heart, tongue, kidney
- **Other meat** – Goat, lamb, veal
- **Cured meat** – Bacon, sausage, ham (choose those that do not contain sugar or nitrates)
- **Nut butter** – Almond butter, macadamia nut butter

Vegetables and Fruits

Vegetables are essential in the keto diet. However, you need to limit intake of those that are high in carbohydrates.

Here are those that should be included in your choices:

- Broccoli
- Cauliflower
- Radishes
- White cabbage
- Green cabbage
- Brussels sprouts
- Zucchini
- Bok choy
- Kale
- Cucumbers
- Olives
- Green beans
- Mushrooms
- Turnips
- Asparagus
- Summer squash
- Bamboo shoots
- Artichoke hearts
- Celery
- Eggplant
- Okra
- Garlic
- Bell pepper

When it comes to fruits, your choices are limited. Fruits are high in sugar, which is the carbohydrate that you'd want to steer clear of when you're on a keto diet.

But you can still eat a few types such as the ones enumerated below:

- Avocado
- Blackberries
- Blueberries
- Raspberries
- Strawberries

Dairy Products

Keto dieters are allowed to consume dairy products, but are encouraged to choose raw and organic products. It's important to choose full fat dairy products over those that are low or free of fat.

Here's a list of the dairy products that you can consume under the keto diet program:

- Greek yogurt
- Heavy whipping cream
- Cream cheese
- Sour cream
- Fresh cream
- Cottage cheese
- Brie
- Mozzarella
- Monterey Jack
- Colby
- Mascarpone
- Cheddar
- Parmesan
- Feta
- Swiss cheese

Nuts and Seeds

Nuts and seeds are a great source of healthy fat and protein. However, they also contain omega 6 fatty acids, so it's imperative not to eat too much of these.

Nuts and seeds allowed on the keto diet:

- Brazil nuts
- Pecans
- Macadamia nuts
- Walnuts
- Almonds
- Hazel nuts
- Pine nuts

Beverages

One of the many things that you have to know about the keto diet is that it is a natural diuretic, which is why dehydration is a common side effect, particularly for those in the initial stage. This makes it imperative to drink at least eight glasses of water a day.

Now what about other drinks and beverages?

Here's a list of what are allowed:

- Broth
- Coffee
-
- Tea
- Coconut milk
- Almond milk

Herbs, Spices, Condiments & Sauces

For most people, this is where things get a little tricky. Many are not aware that some spices actually contain carbs. One may not have any idea that he's loading up on carbs just by spicing up his dish.

Enumerated below are the herbs and spices that you can use while under this diet:

- Basil
- Cayenne pepper
- Cinnamon
- Chili powder
- Oregano
- Cumin
- Parsley
- Thyme
- Rosemary
- Cilantro
- Salt
- Pepper

- Ketchup
- Mustard
- Hot sauce
- Sauerkraut
- Relish
- Mayonnaise
- Horseradish
- Salad dressing
- Worcestershire sauce

Just make sure that the sauces or condiments that you use do not contain any hidden carbohydrates.

Sweeteners

Since sugar is a major no-no in the ketogenic diet program, experts have come up with a list of alternatives that are safe to take in:

- Stevia
- Sucralose
- Erythritol
- Monk fruit
- Swerve

FOODS TO AVOID

As for foods to avoid, you'd want to stay away from the following:

Carbs

Carbohydrates are not allowed in the ketogenic diet for the simple reason that it prevents burning of fat.

Below, you'll find a list of high carb foods that you need to avoid:

- **Grains** – Rice, wheat, barley, oats, rye, corn, quinoa, millet, bulgur, sorghum, amaranth, buckwheat, sprouted grains, and all pasta, breads and crackers made from these grains
- **Beans and legumes** – Kidney beans, chickpeas, lentils, black beans, green peas, lima beans, pinto beans, great northern beans, white beans, black eyed peas, black cannellini beans, fava beans
- **Fruits** – Bananas, apples, pineapple, papaya, oranges, grapes, mangoes, tangerines, all fruit juices, all fruit syrups, all fruit concentrates
- **Starchy vegetables** – Potatoes, sweet potatoes, yams, carrots, peas, yucca, corn, tomatoes
- **Sugars** – Brown sugar, white sugar, cane sugar, raw sugar, honey, agave nectar, maple syrup, turbinado sugar, high fructose corn syrup

Protein

Not all protein sources are to be avoided. In fact, some of them have been listed in the foods that are allowed.

But to make sure you stay in ketosis, do not consume the following:

- Milk and low fat dairy products (low fat yogurt, fat free butter substitute, low fat cream cheese, evaporated skim milk, low fat whipped cream)
- Grain fed meats
- Factory-farmed fish and pork
- Processed meat that contain nitrates

Fats and Oils

It's a must to avoid processed vegetable oils that will not only ruin your diet but also harm your health:

- Soybean oil
- Canola oil
- Corn oil
- Grapeseed oil
- Sunflower oil
- Peanut oil
- Safflower oil
- Sesame oil

Beverages

It's best to keep yourself hydrated with water and other drinks that are keto friendly.

As much as possible, steer clear of the following:

- **Alcohol** – Beers, wines, cocktails, flavored liquers
- **Sugary drinks** – Soda, diet soda, fruit juices, fruit smoothies, coffee or tea with milk or sugar, sweetened milk

Processed food products

Whether you're on the keto diet or not, you should always make it a point to avoid processed foods. These are loaded with chemicals, preservatives, sugars, and trans fats that can harm the health in more ways than one.

Just a few examples of processed food products to avoid include:

- **Commercially baked goods** – Cookies, cakes
- **Sweet treats** – Candies, ice cream
- **Canned goods and instant foods** – Cup noodles, rice packet meals, canned vegetables and meat products
- **"Junk food"** – Potato chips, corn chips, buttered or sweetened popcorn
- **Fast Food** – French fries, burgers, pizza and other foods from fast food chains

Sweeteners

Certain artificial sweeteners have been found to negatively affect blood sugar levels. These include:

- Equal
- Acesulfame
- Aspartame
- Saccharin

Knowing which foods to eat and avoid is one of the first steps towards the ketogenic diet success.

Chapter 6: Tips for Successful Keto Diet

Anyone following the ketogenic diet has one goal in mind: success.

Now, the definition of success can be any of the following:
- Lose a specific amount of weight
- Make a change towards a healthier lifestyle
- Look better and feel better
- Reduce the risk of serious ailments

Success can also mean all of the above! Whatever is your definition of success, allow us to help you get there. Here are some tips that will do just that.

Tip # 1 - Follow the Keto Diet Step by Step

Below, you will find the step by step procedure of the keto diet program. Be sure to follow each step carefully:

Step # 1 – Prepare yourself

It's not only your body that should be prepared for a new diet, but also your mind.
First, you need to set your mind that this is not going to be a walk in the park, that throughout your journey, you will be experiencing numerous hardships and challenges, some of which would even make you want to quit at some point.
If you are prepared for such scenario, it will be so much easier for you to overcome difficulties than if you have no idea of what to expect.
Second, you need to equip yourself with enough knowledge about the ketogenic diet. Yes, this book already provides almost everything you need to know. But there's a plethora of information online about this diet program just in case if you have any more questions. Just make sure that you rely only on reliable sources.
It's also important to prepare not only yourself but also your home and the people around you. Talk to your family about this new diet program you are embarking, as you will need their support and encouragement. Look around your home, particularly your kitchen, and take the time to discard unhealthy food items in there that will tempt you to veer away from the keto diet.

Step # 2 – Measure yourself

Before you can get started with the keto diet, you need to first measure yourself. This will determine your starting point and enable you to track your progress effectively. Here are the stats that you need to know:

- Weight
- Height
- Hips
- Thigh
- Calf
- Wrist
- Forearm

Once you know all these stats, you can use a BMI calculator to find out your BMI and body fat percentage.

Step # 3 – Know the macros

After you've gathered the essential information about your body's current stats, you can go ahead and make use of a keto calculator to determine how many carbohydrates, protein and fat you need to consume to be able to reach the goals that you desire. It's not enough to have a rough idea of these numbers. You need specific figures. Write them down so you don't forget. Generally, experts recommend limiting net carbs to 20 grams and total carbs to 35 grams per day. As for protein, it's good to keep it within 0.6 grams and 0.8 grams per pound lean body mass.

Step # 4 – Plan your meals

The next thing that you have to do is to plan your meals. Write down a weekly menu consisting of dishes that are keto-friendly. In the next chapters of this book, you will find recipes that can help you in your meal planning.

Step # 5 – Monitor your progress

Monitor your progress each week by taking note of the stats that you previously measured in the second step. Keeping a journal will help you track your progress.

TIP # 2 – BE CAREFUL WHEN EATING OUT

For most people, eating out is a break from the chore of cooking and food preparation. It's also bonding time with family or friends. Now that you're on a keto diet, you might be thinking that you will no longer be allowed to dine out. This is not true.

As long as you're careful with your choices not only on food but also on restaurants (and dining partners too), you should not have any problem.

Here are some pointers to remember:

- **Do your research before eating out** – Use the internet to find out the menu of the restaurant you're planning to visit. This way, you can already decide which foods to order when you get there.
- **Eat before leaving the house** – You don't have to eat a full meal but this is just to ensure that you don't arrive at the restaurant too hungry. It's a lot more difficult to stick to your diet when you're very hungry.
- **Go for keto-friendly restaurants** – Some restaurants serve keto-friendly dishes. These include: seafood restaurants, restaurants that serve Greek, Middle Eastern and Mediterranean fare, and grill/barbecue restaurants. It's also a good idea to avoid eating at pizza joints, Italian restaurants, Mexican eateries, sandwich shops and fast food joints.
- **Ask questions** – If you're not sure whether the food you want to order is keto friendly or not, ask the server. For example, you can inquire whether the fish or meat is breaded, or if it comes with high carb sauces or toppings.
- **Dine with the right people** – Don't go out with people who will judge your food choices or make negative comments about your diet. Go out with those who are positive and supportive, and whom you will enjoy dining with.

TIP # 3 - CHANGE YOUR PANTRY

If your pantry is loaded with foods that are not on the "foods to eat" list, you are going to have a harder time sticking to your diet.

Take a good look at your pantry and also your refrigerator and freezer. Let go of all candies, chocolates, ice cream, cereals, crackers, bread and so on. Give food to charity or local food bank.

If this is not possible because there are other people at home who are not using the same diet as you, then it would be best to create a separate pantry or section in the refrigerator for yourself.

Tip # 4 - Read Labels Before Buying

When you're on the keto diet, you need to get better in reading labels. Yes, this can be tricky, as there are plenty terms in those labels that you barely understand. Here are some strategies that can help.

Know the many names of sugar

Sugar comes in many names, and you need to know about all these to ensure that you're not side tracked.

- Brown sugar
- White sugar
- Barley malt syrup
- Agave nectar
- Brown rice syrup
- Beet sugar
- Cane crystals
- Cane juice crystals
- Cane sugar
- Coconut sugar
- Coconut palm sugar
- Dehydrated cane juice
- Invert sugar
- Corn sweetener
- Dextrose
- Dextrin
- Evaporated cane juice
- Fruit juice concentrate
- Fructose
- High-fructose corn syrup
- Glucose
- Honey
- Lactose
- Malt syrup
- Corn syrup
- Corn syrup solids
- Treacle
- Maltodextrin
- Maltose
- Molasses
- Turbinado Sugar
- Maple syrup
- Palm sugar
- Raw sugar
- Xylose
- Rice syrup
- Saccharose
- Sorghum or sorghum syrup
- Syrup
- Sucrose

Be careful of sugar-free labels

Some products are labeled as sugar-free, but would actually contain sugar alcohols, which are just as bad.

Examples of sugar alcohols are:

- Maltitol
- Sorbitol
- Xylitol
- Isomalt
- Hydrogenated starch hydrolysates

Stay away from partially hydrogenated oils

Partially hydrogenated oils are trans fats. Avoid any food product that lists this as one of its ingredients.

TIP # 5 - BUY IN BULK QUANTITIES

Buying in bulk can help you save money when shopping for keto food. But it doesn't mean you have to buy everything in bulk when you go to the grocery.

What you need to do is to plan your menu for the week, and list down all the ingredients that you will be needing. For those that have long shelf life, and those that you will be needing more of, you can buy these in bulk. For example, if most of your dishes require eggs, then you can buy in dozen or in tray instead of per piece.

TIP # 6 - DRINK LOTS OF WATER

As it has been repeated a number of times in this book, drinking water is a must for all keto dieters. Again, this benefits the body in plenty ways.

Since the keto diet is a natural diuretic, doing this will prevent you from getting dehydrated, which is a common side effect of the keto diet. Strive to drink at least eight glasses of water each day.

TIP # 7 - BE AWARE OF ALCOHOL CONSUMPTION

In the previous chapter, it was mentioned that alcohol is not allowed in the keto diet. However, we cannot deny the fact that there would be some people who would not be able to give up alcohol, at least that easily.

Here's a list of a few alcoholic beverages that you can occasionally enjoy while on the keto diet:

- Champagne
- Dry sparkling wine
- Red wine
- White wine
- Whiskey
- Dry martini

These alcoholic beverages are only to be consumed once in a while such as when you're attending a party or going out with your friends. Drink one glass per occasion. Do not consume more than twice a week.

TIP # 8 - DON'T BE AFRAID TO ASK ADVICE

Most of what you need to know to get started and achieve success with the keto diet can be found in this book. However, there may still be areas that we were not able to cover, especially those that are unique to your personal circumstances.

For example, if you have a pre-existing medical condition, it is imperative that you consult a doctor first before starting this diet.

Now if you are unsure of your diet plan, or you are confident with your menu planning skills, do not hesitate to enlist the help of a professional dietician or nutritionist.

TIP # 9 - BE PATIENT AND CONSISTENT

As with any other diet program that's safe and effective, the ketogenic diet does not provide instant success.

Expect that there will be problems, challenges and hurdles along the way. This is why, you need to be patient throughout the journey to be able to reach your goals.

If there are times that you feel like you want to give up, remember your objectives—why you started this in the first place, and for sure, this will give you the motivation you need to go on. Another important virtue is consistency. You will not achieve success in the keto diet if you follow it one day and forget all about it the next day. You need to be consistent and follow the rules to the dot.

TIP # 10 - MAINTAIN A FOOD JOURNAL

Maintaining a food journal makes it easier for you to track your progress, and determine which foods might be hindering your success.

Take note of all the ingredients that you eat during the day, including the portions and sizes. Yes, this takes a lot of time and effort but at some point, you will realize that this makes things a lot easier and more efficient.

Tip # 11 - Use Vitamins and Mineral

Eliminating certain types of foods from your diet will also mean a decline in the vitamins and minerals that you're taking in. To counter the effects of nutritional deficiency, it's a good idea to take the right types of supplements.

Here's a list of the vitamins and minerals that you should consider taking a supplement of:

- **Sodium** – 3,000 to 5,000 mg per day
- **Potassium** – 3,000 mg per day
- **Magnesium** – 500 mg per day
- **Calcium** – 1,000 to 1,200 mg per day
- **Vitamin D** – 1,000 IU for every 25 pounds of body weight
- **Vitamin A** – 0.7 to 0.9 mg per day
- **Omega 3 fatty acids** – 3000 mg fish oil per day

Tip # 12 - Join Social Groups

Expect to experience numerous challenges and problems during your ketogenic journey. One of the things that can help is joining social groups.

When you join social groups, whether online or offline, you're going to meet other people who are experiencing the same challenges as you, and who are going through their own pains and hardships. This will make you feel that you are not alone in this journey.

Also, in these social groups, you will find many inspiring success stories that will show you that this is doable. It will make you see that if others can do it, so can you.

Here are a few examples of social groups that you can join online:

- Ketosis & The Ketogenic Community
- Ketogenic Diet (Recipes & Meal Prep)
- Ketogenic Lifestyle
- Ketogenic Diet for Beginners

Tip # 13 - Manage Social Outings

Eating out in restaurants is not the only challenge for the keto dieter. There are many social functions and gatherings that will prove to be a challenge as well.

If you're a keto dieter attending a social gathering, and you keep refusing foods that are being served to you, the host (and other guests) will think that you're either rude or weird.

So this doesn't happen, here are what you can do:

- **Explain to the hosts your situation** – When you confirm your attendance to the hosts, inform them that you've just started out on a ketogenic diet. This way, they won't be surprised (or offended) when they see that you now have different food preferences.
- **Eat a snack before going to the party** – This will prevent you from overeating, and still allow you to enjoy the gathering.
- **Focus on other activities** – The food is only one part of the party. There are many activities that you can do there aside from filling yourself with food. Mingle with other guests, catch up with friends you haven't seen for a long time, strut your stuff on the dance floor, engage in the activities available, and so on.
- **Skip the event** – If you are not comfortable going to the event for whatever reason that you have, you don't have to force yourself.

Tip # 14 - Come Up with a Suitable Reward System

Many things can cause you to lose motivation and get sidetracked during your diet. But if you come up with a reward system, you will be able to get that motivation back.

First, you need to establish tangible goals. Then for each goal that you accomplish, reward yourself with something that you want so badly.

The reward can be a new book that you've been wanting to read or a movie date with your friends. It should not be food-related as this will defeat the purpose of your dieting.

CHAPTER 7: DOS AND DON'TS OF KETO DIET

Learning about what you should and should not do on a keto diet can spell difference between getting results and falling off track. So keep this list in mind, as it is sure to come in handy at one point in your journey to a keto lifestyle.

DO INCREASE PROTEIN INTAKE

Since the keto diet is low-carb, your body needs to get energy in another way. This is where protein comes in. By increasing your protein intake, your body is able to break down proteins for energy.

To get enough protein, make sure two or three of your daily meals include one or more high-quality protein sources.

Your best options for minimal fat and calorie are poultry, beef, pork, offal, fish and shellfish. So make room in your diet for white-meat chicken, duck, pheasant, quail, ground beef or pork, steak, pork chops, ham, tenderloin, goat, veal and turkey. Get your seafood fix with wild-caught cod, halibut, salmon, trout, tuna, snapper, mahi-mahi, flounder, mackerel, catfish, clams, crab, lobster, mussels, oysters, squid and scallops. Try out organ meats like tongue, kidney, liver and heart.

You could also add egg whites to your meals. Or whip up a sauce or dressing or even a shake and then mix in low-carb, unflavored protein powder.

If your meals need some extra fat, you can get protein from bacon and sausage (should not be cured in sugar), whole eggs (preferably free-range), high-protein cheese (cheddar, mozzarella and parmesan) and nut butters (almond, macadamia and peanut).

Just don't overdo it. The recommended levels per pound of lean body mass vary depending on your lifestyle or goal: 0.6g to 0.8g if you're sedentary, 0.8g to 1.0g if you're active, and 1.0g to 1.2g if muscle gain is a priority.

DO INCREASE SODIUM INTAKE

With salt, less is not always better. If you were on a high-carb diet, then yes, you need to minimize your intake. But with a low-carb program such as the keto diet, you actually need to up your salt intake.

For one, your body will be excreting more salt. And you will be cutting out sodium-processed foods.

Low blood sodium levels can hamper a number of physiological functions. It could, for instance, lead to electrolyte imbalance, which many believe is the culprit behind keto flu. Keto flu is a condition common among those who transition to a keto diet, and typical symptoms include headaches, light-headedness, fatigue and in some cases constipation.

To avoid or counteract this, it is important to replenish the sodium that your body loses with extra salt. The target, according to some experts, is 2g to 4g of sodium per day.

The simplest way to go about this is by incorporating more salt in your food, manually or through salted butter or bullion. You can, for instance, sprinkle Himalayan sea salt (also called pink salt) on your meals or even in your water.

It also helps to drink a cup of organic bone broth daily, eat sodium-rich vegetables such as celery and cucumbers, munch on salted macadamia nuts, or have bacon for breakfast.

DO LEARN FROM SUCCESSFUL KETO DIETERS

To increase your chances of pulling it off, consider reading up on keto-diet success stories or on guides from those who have "been there, done that."

This kind of research can help you start off on the right track, if you're a newbie, or stay on track, if you're struggling because you aren't seeing results or are finding it hard to adjust and cope with the changes.

Through first-hand accounts of keto dieters, you can learn what it's really like to make the switch. And you can prepare for the challenges that lie ahead along with the demands of the diet.

Looking into how the diet worked for others, and how their lives have changed for the better, can also provide you the inspiration and motivation you need to keep going, in case you're thinking about giving up.

Plus, their practical tips are almost always worth a try. You can find everything from how to avoid the usual pitfalls to tricks for curbing cravings to tried-and-tested recipes and the most keto-friendly products.

Who else would tell you that Omega-3 is a must, that cast-iron pans make for tastier meals, that lemon water comes in handy, that dark chocolate chips can save the day, and that toasted coconut flakes could be your go-to cereal? Keto-fans may just hold the answers.

DO TRACK YOUR PROGRESS

There are different methods to track your progress on a keto diet.

One is to keep a journal of your keto journey. Take notes daily or at least on a regular basis. Write about the dietary changes you made and how you are feeling—physically and mentally.

You can even rate your mood, mental clarity or energy on a scale of 1 to 10. And don't forget to record your ketone levels and any specific results in terms of your weight and body measurements. All this can help you (and any healthcare professional you're consulting with) figure out what works best for you.

Take measurements of your bust, calves, hips, thighs and waist at the beginning and end of each month. This may be more effective and accurate than the scale, as you could be losing fat and inches but not dropping the pounds.

You can also try on clothes that fit you tightly before you began the diet or check a few weeks after if you are a size smaller, garment-wise.

Or you could pose in the same clothing and angle for before-and-after photos: the "before" photo on day one and the "after" photos on days 20, 40 and 60.

And if you want to monitor metrics, invest in a body-fat analyzer. You can use this and a corresponding app to conduct regular hydrostatic body-fat testing and to track everything from your body weight, fat, water and mass to your BMI, protein level, BMR and metabolic age.

DO KEEP YOUR BODY HYDRATED

With the keto diet, you need to make a conscious effort to stay hydrated.

The keto diet has a natural diuretic effect, with your body excreting more water than it normally does. So you end up losing lots of electrolytes and fluid, especially when you're starting out.

If you don't replenish those electrolytes and drink up, dehydration follows and could result in keto flu. It could also impede your progress since your body will be storing as much fat as it can.

Your best source of hydration is water, plenty of it. Still or sparkling water is fine. What's important is that you drink water constantly so that you drink almost a gallon a day or at least the amount (ounces) that is equivalent to half your body weight (pounds). Adding a squeeze of lime, orange or lemon helps, if you prefer your water flavored. And if you find yourself sweating extra due to the heat or post-workout, make sure to drink even more.

Your other options include chicken or bone broth (rich in nutrients and vitamins and can be very energizing), coffee and herbal tea (black or green), coconut or almond milk (unsweetened), and sports drinks (with stevia or sucralose).

DON'T EAT FAST FOOD

Steer clear of fast food as much as possible. While you can eat out and still stick to your diet, you need to mindful about where you dine.

Fast-food outlets are notorious for serving food with plenty of preservatives and chemicals. You could order a burger without the bun, but the burger patty may still contain fillers and added salts.

Sometimes even their "healthy" dishes have hidden carbs and sugars. The salads, for instance, usually use refined sugar and unsaturated oils. Plus, a restaurant's definition of healthy rarely matches what is considered healthy under a keto diet.

Eating out might feel like your reward after days of strict keto dieting. But if you don't choose restaurants carefully, it could set you back and all your hard work might go to waste.

The good news is that there chains that cater to low-carb diets. You could ask if they have keto-friendly meat options or request for extra vegetables in place of a high-carb food item.

Or you could search for an all-vegan restaurant that offers more choices that will keep you on track. Just don't hesitate to ask questions if you are unsure about the food sources or want to know more about a dish's ingredients.

You will need to dine out at some point in your keto journey. Just don't risk your chance of success with fast food, especially when there are other alternatives.

DON'T FEAR FAT

Shying or staying away from fats may feel like the right thing to do when you want to lose weight. But in a keto diet, you actually need fats.

The keto diet is largely fats, with fats accounting for 75 percent of food sources—healthy fats that is. Yes, as long as they're the good kind, fats can boost your energy, help you think clearly and bring you closer to your goal.

The recommend amount is three to four tablespoons of fat per meal.

Among your options are animal fats like bacon, unsalted butter, cheese, ghee, heavy cream and mayonnaise. If there are versions derived from grass-fed animals, go with those.

Plant-based saturated fats work well too, with the list including avocado oil, coconut oil, extra virgin olive oil, MCT oil and vegan mayonnaise.

You can cook with these delicious fats or add them as flavoring or dressing.

Also, when you're buying meat, select fattier cuts of steak, roasts, tenderloin, ham, pork chops, goat, turkey, veal and lamb. Fattier is likewise better when it comes to fish.

And if you are a fan of fresh fruit, make avocados a big part of your diet. These are low-carb and bursting in healthy fats, and you can use them in a variety of recipes.

DON'T INCREASE CARB INTAKE

Your carb intake should be limited when you're on the keto diet. So it's important to measure and monitor just how much carbohydrates you are consuming every day.

The keto carb limit is said to be from 35g to 50g of total carbs per day, although some advocates believe as few as 20 grams daily is ideal.

In terms of net carbs, the recommended limit is generally between 20g and 30g. Net carbs, computed by deducting the grams of total fiber from grams of total carbs, are what most keto dieters use to count carbs.

To stay in ketosis, you need to watch your carb intake and ensure it doesn't go beyond this limit.

So keep an eye out for food with hidden carbs. Examples include breaded meats, chicken wings (with barbecue or buffalo sauce), low-fat yogurt and milk.

You also need to eliminate high-carb sources from your diet, particularly sugary and starchy food such as rice, pasta and bread.

Instead, focus on low-carb alternatives that you can consume many times each day. With vegetables, anything besides corn, large tomatoes and potatoes is acceptable. You can have keto-friendly vegetables multiple times each day along with avocado and nuts.

DON'T CONSUME MANY ROOT VEGETABLES

Vegetables that grow underground are rich in fiber and vitamins A and C. But because some of them are too starchy and carb-heavy, you need to choose your root vegetables carefully and consume them in moderation. Otherwise, with all the glucose being broken down, your body will continue to be a sugar burner and you risk ruining your keto diet.

For starters, cross off the usual suspects—regular and sweet potatoes—from the list. One cup of potatoes contains about 26g of carbs.

Then take note of the root veggies that many do not realize are high in carbs as well: beets, carrots, cassava, Jerusalem artichoke, parsnips, yams and yucca. A one-cup serving of parsnips has 24g of carbs, beets 24g, and carrots 12g.

As for the ones that are not as high-carb but should be eaten occasionally only, you have garlic, onion, spring onion, leek, mushrooms, radishes and winter squash.

Most of these can be used as flavoring (such as onion for soup), so it should be easy to track your consumption and avoid going overboard. But of course, it also helps to pay attention to the number of carbs a particular vegetable has before your incorporate it into your program.

DON'T EXERCISE DURING THE FIRST TWO WEEKS

The first two weeks are a tough time for every keto dieter. This period can take a toll on your body, with some suffering from keto flu.

If you don't exercise regularly but would like to start now that you're on a keto diet, hold it off until after the first two weeks. You won't feel like exercising anyway. With all the changes your body is adapting to, you might actually be too weak to work out.

So slow down and focus on getting through this rough patch. After your body becomes fat-adapted, you might feel more energized and motivated to get back on your feet and become more active. Plus, now that your body is producing ketones efficiently, you can look forward to increased strength, muscle gains and fat loss.

You could, for instance, try high-intensity aerobic exercises. With such routines, your body will be tapping fat as its primary energy source (since carbohydrates are not available). And you can reap the benefits after your first two weeks on this diet.

Of course, there are other types of workouts that suit keto dieters. Just remember not to push too early and too hard. Taking things in stages is a smart move as is sticking to what you feel comfortable with.

CHAPTER 8: FREQUENTLY ASKED QUESTIONS

WHY DOES THE KETO DIET HELP YOU TO LOSE WEIGHT FASTER THAN OTHER DIETS?

With the keto diet, your weight will drop quickly the first week. The usual weight loss during this adjustment phase is from 2 to 7 pounds, although some lose up to 10 pounds.

Most of that will be water weight. This is because your body, in response to your reduced carb intake, won't burn fat right away. Instead it will start by burning all your glycogen reserves. Between 2g and 3g of water is bound to each gram of glycogen, making for drastic water-weight loss. Plus, after your glycogen reserves are depleted, water required to store glycogen is eliminated.

Your body will then transition into a fat-burning mode, and for the second to fourth weeks you can expect to lose one to two pounds per week.

This is referred to as the adaptation phase, as your body is getting used to tapping fat—instead of carbs—as your main fuel source.

For regular and stable weight loss, you need to keep your daily net carb intake below 20g and monitor your calories.

It also helps that there's more fat and protein than carbs in your body. Fat and protein leave you feeling full longer than carbs do, so you won't be hungry as often.

By the fourth week or so, you will be fat-adapted and can continue to loss one to two pounds each week, depending on the calories you consume and how much physical activity you engage in. At this point, you probably won't have carb cravings anymore and your improved energy will allow you to step up your workouts.

Just keep in mind that the rate and amount of weight loss vary with each person and is determined by a range of factors, including your age, metabolism, activity level, how much body fat you have and how committed you are to the keto diet.

WHAT SHOULD I DO BEFORE FOLLOWING THE KETO DIET?

Here are some ways you can prepare for and successfully ease into the keto diet.

Do your homework

Read up on the keto diet. There are tons on online articles and guides that you can easily access plus a number of books that make for great reference materials.

Your research should cover the basics of the keto diet—what it is, what it's like, what it requires, what you can expect. Also look up recommended foods, keto-friendly alternatives for your favorites, and tried-and-tested recipes and meal plans.

Do the math

To be able to reach and maintain ketosis, you need to restrict your net carb intake. And to be able to choose foods that will keep you within your limit, you need to learn how to calculate net carbs early on.

The net carb equation is pretty simple. It involves just two values: total carbohydrate and dietary fiber. Both these appear on standard U.S. nutrition labels.

To determine a food item's net carb content (per serving), just subtract the dietary fiber content from the total carbohydrate content.

If the number of grams you get is too close to, exceeds or is more than half of your net carb limit, then it's not keto-friendly.

Clear your kitchen

Check your refrigerator and pantry for non-ketogenic foods and keep them out of reach. You'll have hard-to-resist carb cravings when you start out, and you might be tempted to give into those cravings if you can easily get your hands on bread, chips, pasta, cereal, corn, rice, cookies, ice cream, chocolate, candy, honey, maple syrup and sugary drinks.

In addition to these, you need to steer clear of beans, apples, oranges, bananas, yams and potatoes, as these are all carb-heavy.

Stock up

Shop for and fill your kitchen with food that's keto-friendly. Begin with the staples: butter, coconut oil, fatty meats (beef, fish, pork and poultry), eggs, leafy greens and other low-carb vegetables (cauliflower, broccoli).

Also get some fruits (avocados, blackberries, raspberries), nuts and seeds (walnuts, macadamias, sunflower seeds), kale chips, high-fat salad dressing and cream, and hard cheeses. It pays to have sweeteners (monk fruit, erythritol, stevia) too, as these will help keep you away from bread and sugary items.

Remember to hit the aisles only after eating a small fatty meal. Being satiated, rather than starved, in a grocery store reduces the likelihood that you would buy something that's not on your list. Or simply shop online instead.

To prevent overeating and keep your calorie count low, go for less variety in terms of the foods you stock at a given time. Also, store your favorites in places that are not quickly accessible or within view.

Plan meals

Well-planned meals will set you off on the right track, and you won't have to waste time worrying or stressing about what to have for your next meal.

The key to successful meal planning: your macros. You need to have the right ratio of fats (75 percent), protein (20 percent) and carbs (5 percent) every day, and you can use online macro calculators to determine the required number of grams for each.

Search for recipes based on your calculations and prepare your week's meal plan accordingly.

Make small changes

Prepare for the demands of the keto diet by gradually reducing carbs and increasing fats.
- When you dine out, skip the burger bun and have it replaced with lettuce. And instead of having rice or potatoes with your meal, request for green veggies.
- Use more oil when you cook.
- Add salt to your meals.
- Begin taking supplements (mainly for magnesium, potassium and sodium).

Tell your family and friends

Explain to your loved ones what the keto diet is all about, why you want to try it, and how this will change your meals and eating habits. This way, they can provide you support rather than set you back.

Choose a start date

The date should be on a week where your schedule is clear—no deadlines to beat, no obligations to attend to, no planned trips, parties or lunch/dinner dates. The whole week has to be non-stressful so you can rest well during the adjustment phase.

SHOULD I HAVE A LIFELONG KETO DIET?

While the keto diet has grown popular in recent years, there aren't research studies yet that support its effectiveness as a lifelong diet.

But many believe it is a short-term fix, a temporary diet you go on for four to six months if your primary goal is weight control. The good news is you can expect sustained fat loss. If you are able to maintain healthy eating habits, chances are you won't regain the weight you lost. Some advocates feel staying on the keto diet is beneficial if you have diabetes, anxiety and neurological disorders, commonly experience brain fog, or need the continued energy boost.

CAN I HAVE KETO DIET IF I AM IN VEGETARIAN DIET?

Yes. The keto diet can be adapted to fit a vegetarian's lifestyle. This version, referred to as the vegetarian ketogenic diet, is designed around plant-based meals but incorporates principles of the keto diet. So it lets vegetarians enjoy the health benefits of ketosis without drastically changing their lifestyle.

The vegetarian ketogenic diet excludes all kinds of animal flesh: meat, poultry and fish. The only animal products allowed are eggs and dairy.

The list of acceptable foods also includes non-starchy vegetables like leafy greens, low-sugar fruits, healthy fats, and plant-based proteins such as nuts, seeds, nutritional yeast, tempeh, spirulina and natto.

CHAPTER 9: WHY USE INSTANT POT COOKING?

So far, we've covered almost everything there is to know about the ketogenic diet. But before we get to the cooking part, let's first get to know more about this versatile device that we are going to use for whipping up delicious dishes.

WHAT IS AN INSTANT POT?

The Instant Pot is a versatile kitchen device that acts as a multi-cooker. It can function as a slow cooker, pressure cooker, rice cooker, steamer, warmer, and more.
You can use it to sear, brown and sauté food, as well as bake breads and pastries. It can even be used to make yogurt. That's how versatile and convenient this kitchen tool is.

HOW DOES IT WORK?

The Instant Pot has several functions but it works primarily as a pressure cooker.
During this process, the liquid inside the pot is used to create steam and increase pressure. The pressure boils the liquid and cooks the food at a faster rate while retaining the nutrients and flavor.

WHAT ARE THE SPECIAL BUTTONS AND FEATURES?

When you look at the Instant Pot, you will see that it has many buttons indicating different cooking methods. Each button has a pre-set cooking time and pressure setting.

Button	Pressure Setting	Cook Time
Slow cook	Normal	4 Hours
Pressure	Low, High	Manual
Soup	High	30 minutes
Stew/Meat	High	35 minutes
Bean/Chili	High	30 minutes
Poultry	High	15 minutes
Rice	Low	Automatic
Multigrain	High	40 minutes
Porridge	High	20 minutes

Steam	High	10 minutes
Yogurt	3 programs	Manual
Sauté	Normal	Manual
Manual	Defaults to High but can be adjusted	Manual
Adjust	-	-
Timer	-	Manual
Keep warm/Cancel	-	Manual

For some buttons, there are pre-set cooking times but for others such as pressure cooking, you will need to manually enter how long you want the food to be cooked.

When it comes to releasing the pressure, there are two ways to do this: the **quick release method** and the **natural release method**.

In the quick release method, you need to turn the steam release valve to venting position. It takes about one to two minutes for the quick release pressure to complete. This method is ideal for foods that you do not want to overcook such as vegetables or salmon. This is not advisable for dishes with high starch content.

In the natural release method, you let the pot depressurize by itself. This takes about 10 to 30 minutes. The amount of time primarily depends on the amount of the cooking liquid inside the pot. This is best used for dishes with plenty liquid or those that are foamy.

It's imperative to wait for all the steam to be released before uncovering the pot. Opening the pot before all steam has been released can be dangerous.

How to Use it Effectively

To use the Instant Pot effectively, of course, you need to first read the manual carefully and understand how the whole process works.

For best results, here are some more tips to follow:

- **Plan the meal preparation** – Read the recipe that you're using and prepare everything that's required. Aside from the ingredients, some recipes call for use of baking pans or steamer racks. Make sure that these devices fit inside your Instant Pot.
- **Use plenty cooking liquid** – This is especially true if you are pressure cooking. Plenty liquid is needed to build up steam and pressure, and for your food to cook evenly.
- **Slice food into smaller pieces** – This will cook your food more evenly and more quickly.
- **Do not overfill the pot** – If you do, the food will not be cooked evenly.

- **Brown and sauté before pressure cooking** – In most recipes that you'll find in the next chapter, you'll see that the meat or poultry will need to be browned or sautéed first. This takes more time but it locks in more flavor.

TIPS AND CAUTIONS OF INSTANT POT USAGE

Aside from effective cooking, it's also important to learn how to use the Instant Pot safely. Here are some safety tips you can't afford to ignore:

- **Do not open the pot until all steam has been released** – Use either the quick release method or natural release method discussed earlier for depressurizing the pot first before opening.
- **Do not leave the Instant Pot alone** – Don't make the mistake of leaving your Instant Pot unsupervised while cooking. Yes, it does its job mostly on its own but you need to be there for safety purposes.
- **Do not use the Instant Pot for pressure frying** – This is not safe. The Instant Pot does not work as a commercial pressure fryer.

COOKING TIMETABLE OF VARIOUS FOODS

Most recipes indicate the amount of time necessary for cooking foods in the Instant Pot. But just so you have an idea, here's the cooking time table for various foods.

Food	Cooking Time for Fresh	Cooking Time for Frozen
Whole crab	2 to 3 minutes	4 to 5 minutes
Whole fish	4 to 5 minutes	5 to 7 minutes
Fish fillet	2 to 3 minutes	3 to 4 minutes
Fish steak	3 to 4 minutes	4 to 6 minutes
Lobster	2 to 3 minutes	3 to 4 minutes
Mussels	1 to 2 minutes	2 to 3 minutes
Shrimp/Prawn	1 to 3 minutes	2 to 4 minutes
Beef/Stew meat	20 minutes per 1 lb.	
Meat ball	5 minutes per 1 lb.	
Dressed beef	25 minutes per 1 lb.	
Beef small slices	15 minutes per 1 lb.	
Beef big slices	25 minutes per 1 lb.	
Beef ribs	20 to 25 minutes	
Beef shank	25 to 30 minutes	

Beef oxtail	40 to 50 minutes	
Chicken breast	6 to 8 minutes	
Whole chicken	8 minutes per 1 lb.	
Chicken, sliced	10 to 15 minutes	
Duck, sliced	12 to 15 minutes	
Whole duck	15 minutes per 1 lb.	
Ham, sliced	9 to 12 minutes	
Ham shoulder	8 minutes per 1 lb.	
Lamb, cubed	10 to 15 minutes	
Lamb stew meat	12 to 15 minutes	
Lamb leg	15 minutes per 1 lb.	
Pork loin roast	20 minutes per 1 lb.	
Pork butt roast	15 minutes per 1 lb.	
Turkey breast	7 to 9 minutes	
Turkey leg	15 to 20 minutes	
Veal chops	5 to 8 minutes	
Veal roast	12 minutes per 1 lb.	
Whole quail	8 minutes per 1 lb.	
Artichoke heart	4 to 5 minutes	5 to 6 minutes
Whole artichoke	9 to 11 minutes	11 to 13 minutes
Asparagus	1 to 2 minutes	2 to 3 minutes
Green beans	1 to 2 minutes	2 to 3 minutes
Beetroot	11 to 13 minutes	13 to 15 minutes
Broccoli florets	1 to 2 minutes	2 to 3 minutes
Broccoli stalks	3 to 4 minutes	4 to 5 minutes
Brussels sprout	2 to 3 minutes	3 to 4 minutes
Cabbage	3 to 4 minutes	4 to 5 minutes
Carrot, sliced	2 to 3 minutes	3 to 4 minutes
Cauliflower	2 to 3 minutes	3 to 4 minutes
Celery chunks	2 to 3 minutes	3 to 4 minutes
Collard greens	4 to 5 minutes	3 to 4 minutes
Corn kernels	1 to 2 minutes	2 to 3 minutes
Corn on the cob	3 to 5 minutes	4 to 6 minutes
Eggplant slices	3 to 4 minutes	4 to 5 minutes
Green beans	2 to 3 minutes	3 to 4 minutes
Leafy greens	4 to 5 minutes	5 to 6 minutes
Leeks	2 to 3 minutes	3 to 4 minutes
Mixed veggies	3 to 4 minutes	4 to 6 minutes

Okra	2 to 3 minutes	3 to 4 minutes
Onion	2 to 3 minutes	3 to 4 minutes
Parsnip	3 to 4 minutes	4 to 5 minutes
Peas	1 to 2 minutes	2 to 3 minutes
Potatoes	3 to 4 minutes	4 to 5 minutes
Pumpkin	4 to 5 minutes	6 to 7 minutes
Spinach	1 to 2 minutes	2 to 3 minutes
Sweet potato	2 to 4 minutes	4 to 6 minutes
Tomatoes	2 to 3 minutes	4 to 5 minutes

FREQUENTLY ASKED QUESTIONS

FAQ # 1 – Why is it necessary to conduct an initial test run?

An initial test run is necessary so that the user will become familiar with how the Instant Pot works. At the same time, it shows you if the device is working properly.

FAQ # 2 – Can you burn food with the Instant Pot?

The good news is, you can't. Most cooking programs have pre-set cooking times. The pot will automatically stop cooking once the cooking duration is over.

For manual cooking methods, the device comes with a burn protection mechanism that halts heating to avoid burning the food. Still, it's important not to leave the cooking unattended, especially if using the sauté mode.

FAQ # 3 – Is the Instant Pot dishwasher safe?

Most of the components are dishwasher safe. These include the inner pot, glass lid, steam rack, rice paddle, and pressure cooker lid. However, you cannot submerge in water the housing that contains the electronic components.

FAQ # 4 – Why does the Instant Pot make clicking noise? Should this be a cause for concern?

This is normal and indicates that the Instant Pot is working. You should not be worried if you hear a clicking sound while using this device.

FAQ # 5 –What is the minimum amount of liquid to be used?

The minimum amount of liquid required is 1 cup to 2 cups.

FAQ # 6 – Why is the steam release handle loose?

This is a safety feature that lets the pressure to be released manually, which is why it is wobbly and loose.

Chapter 10: 5 Keto Diet Appetizer Recipes

1. Artichokes with Avocado Dip

Serves: 2
Preparation time: 20 minutes
Ingredients:

1 onion, sliced into wedges
1 tablespoon lemon zest
2 whole artichokes, trimmed and sliced in half
1 avocado
1 tablespoon lemon juice
3 tablespoons coconut cream
1 teaspoon salt

Preparation:

1) Place a steamer basket inside the Instant Pot.
2) Pour in 2 cups of water to the pot.
3) Press the sauté button.
4) Bring water to a boil.
5) Add the onion and lemon zest to the water.
6) Place the artichokes on top of the rack.
7) Cover the pot.
8) Choose manual setting.
9) Cook at high pressure for 8 minutes.
10) Do a quick pressure release.
11) In a food processor, blend the rest of the ingredients.
12) Serve the artichokes with the blended dip.

Serving Suggestion: You can also serve this with other vegetables such as zucchini sticks.
Tip: To test for doneness, pinch the artichoke leaves and see if tender enough.

Nutritional Information Per Serving:

Calories   380
Total Fat 30.3g
Saturated Fat 7.9g
Cholesterol 0mg
Sodium 1290mg
Total Carbohydrate 8.6g
Dietary Fiber 6.5g
Total Sugars 3.1g
Protein 6.9g
Potassium 632mg

2. CHICKEN BRUSCHETTA

Serves: 8

Preparation time: 30 minutes

Ingredients:

1 ¼ lb. chicken breast (boneless and skinless)

1 cup enchilada sauce

Salt and pepper to taste

8 oz. cream cheese

8 slices almond flour bread

Preparation:

1) Put the chicken breast inside the Instant Pot.
2) Pour the enchilada sauce on top of the chicken.
3) Season with the salt and pepper.
4) Secure the pot.
5) Select manual function.
6) Cook at high pressure for 12 minutes.
7) Release the pressure naturally.
8) Stir in the cream cheese.
9) Shred the chicken with 2 forks.
10) Spread the chicken and sauce on each bread slice.

Serving Suggestion: Top with avocado cubes and parsley.

Tip: You can also make use of other keto bread substitutes such as coconut flour bread and cloud bread.

Nutritional Information Per Serving:

Calories 282

Total Fat 29g

Saturated Fat 12g

Cholesterol 76mg

Sodium 594mg

Total Carbohydrates 14g

Sugars 1g

Protein 19g

Potassium 335mg

3. BUTTERED MUSHROOMS

Serves: 4
Preparation time: 25 minutes
Ingredients:

4 tablespoons butter

4 cups white mushrooms

3 cloves garlic, crushed and minced

½ cup fresh parsley, chopped and divided

4 sprigs fresh oregano, chopped

4 sprigs fresh thyme, chopped

1 cup vegetable broth

Salt and pepper to taste

Preparation:

1) Select the sauté function in the Instant Pot.
2) Add the butter.
3) Add the mushrooms and garlic.
4) Cook for 3-5 minutes.
5) Set aside 3 tablespoons parsley.
6) Place the rest of the parsley, oregano and thyme in the pot.
7) Stir well.
8) Pour in the broth.
9) Season with the salt and pepper.
10) Cover the pot.
11) Set it to manual mode.
12) Cook at high pressure for 5 minutes.
13) Release the pressure quickly.
14) Press sauté.
15) Simmer until sauce has thickened.

Serving Suggestion: Garnish with the remaining parsley.

Tip: Choose big sized mushrooms for this dish.

Nutritional Information Per Serving:

Calories   140

Total Fat 16.4g

Saturated Fat 9.5g

Cholesterol 31mg

Sodium 282mg

Total Carbohydrate 4.4g

Dietary Fiber 2g

Total Sugars 1.5g

Protein 4.2g

Potassium 362mg

4. BACON WRAPPED ASPARAGUS

Serves: 6
Preparation time: 10 minutes
Ingredients:
1 lb. asparagus spears, sliced in half
8 oz. bacon slices
Preparation:
1) Add 2 cups of water to the Instant Pot.
2) Wrap 3-4 asparagus spears with a bacon slice.
3) Place a steamer rack inside the pot.
4) Put the wrapped asparagus on top of the rack.
5) Cover the pot.
6) Choose manual setting.
7) Cook at high pressure for 3 minutes.
8) Release the pressure naturally.

Serving Suggestion: Serve with a dipping sauce mixture of mayo and mustard.
Tip: You can also wrap fried bacon around the asparagus if you like.
Nutritional Information Per Serving:
Calories   358
Total Fat 26.6g
Saturated Fat 8.7g
Cholesterol 70mg
Sodium 1464mg
Total Carbohydrate 3.8g
Dietary Fiber 1.6g
Total Sugars 1.4g
Protein 25.1g
Potassium 511mg

5. Hot Onion Dip

Serves: 8
Preparation time: 30 minutes
Ingredients:
1 cup onion, grated
8 oz. cream cheese
1 cup full fat mayo
1 cup Swiss cheese, grated
Preparation:
1) Combine all the ingredients in a baking dish.
2) Cover the dish with foil.
3) Pour 1 cup of water into the Instant Pot.
4) Place a steamer rack inside the pot.
5) Put the baking dish on top of the rack.
6) Cover the pot.
7) Set it to manual.
8) Cook at high pressure for 15 minutes.
9) Release the pressure naturally.

Serving Suggestion: Serve with vegetable sticks, pork rinds or low carb crackers.
Tip: You can also blend the ingredients in a food processor to shorten preparation time.
Nutritional Information Per Serving:
Calories   271
Total Fat 23.5g
Saturated Fat 10.1g
Cholesterol 51mg
Sodium 319mg
Total Carbohydrate 6.8g
Dietary Fiber 0.3g
Total Sugars 2.7g
Protein 6.2g
Potassium 68mg

CHAPTER 11: 15 KETO DIET BREAKFAST RECIPES

6. BREAKFAST CASSEROLE

Serves: 6
Preparation time: 50 minutes
Ingredients:

Cooking spray

2 tablespoons avocado oil

6 oz. breakfast sausage

1 ½ cups broccoli, grated

2 cloves garlic, minced

Salt and pepper to taste

6 eggs

¼ cup heavy cream

1 cup Monterey Jack cheese, shredded

1 stalk green onion, sliced

1 avocado, sliced

Preparation:

1) Coat a soufflé dish with cooking spray. Choose the sauté setting.
2) Pour in the avocado oil. Add the sausage and cook for 4 minutes.
3) Add the grated broccoli and garlic. Season with the salt and pepper.
4) Cook for 2 minutes.
5) Transfer to the soufflé dish.
6) In a bowl, beat the eggs.
7) Stir in the cream, green onion and cheese.
8) Pour this on top of the sausage mixture. Cover the dish with foil.
9) Add 1 cup of water into the Instant Pot.
10) Place a steamer rack inside the pot. Seal the pot. Select manual mode.
11) Cook at high pressure for 35 minutes. Release the pressure naturally.

Serving Suggestion: Top the casserole with sliced avocado or salsa.

Tip: You can also use other types of cheese like mozzarella or cheddar.

Nutritional Information Per Serving:

Calories   351

Total Fat 32.2g

Saturated Fat 14.2g

Cholesterol 211mg

Sodium 387mg

Total Carbohydrate 5.2g

Dietary Fiber 2.1g

Total Sugars 1g

Protein 17.2g

Potassium 415mg

7. Bacon & Egg Quiche

Serves: 4
Preparation time: 20 minutes
Ingredients:

8 slices bacon, chopped

4 eggs

1 ½ cups heavy whipping cream

¼ teaspoon nutmeg

Salt and pepper to taste

1 1/3 cup Swiss cheese, shredded and divided

Preparation:

1) Select the sauté setting in the Instant Pot.
2) Cook the bacon until golden crisp.
3) Drain on a paper towel.
4) In a bowl, beat the eggs, cream, nutmeg, salt and pepper.
5) Coat the inside of a baking pan.
6) Layer it with shredded cheese.
7) Add another layer, this time of the cooked bacon.
8) Pour on top of the bacon and cheese the egg mixture.
9) Place a steamer rack inside the pot.
10) Put the baking pan on top of the rack.
11) Cover the pot.
12) Set it to manual.
13) Cook at high pressure for 25 minutes.
14) Release the pressure quickly.
15) Top with the remaining cheese.
16) Wait for 10 minutes until the cheese has melted.
17) Flip onto a serving plate.

Serving Suggestion: Sprinkle chopped green onion on top as garnish.

Tip: Use bacon strips instead of chopped bacon if you'd like a richer flavour.

Nutritional Information Per Serving:

Calories   570

Total Fat 47.6g

Saturated Fat 23.6g

Cholesterol 323mg

Sodium 1034mg

Total Carbohydrate 4.2g

Dietary Fiber 0g

Total Sugars 1g

Protein 31g

Potassium 344mg

8. EGG CUPS

Serves: 4
Preparation time: 15 minutes
Ingredients:

4 eggs
1 cup onion, diced
1 cup bell pepper, diced
1 cup mushrooms, diced
1 cup tomatoes, diced

½ cup cheddar cheese, shredded
¼ cup half and half
Salt and pepper to taste
2 tablespoons cilantro, chopped

Preparation:

1) Combine all the ingredients in a bowl.
2) Divide the mixture into 4 glass jars.
3) Put on the lids but do not close tightly.
4) Pour 2 cups of water into the Instant Pot.
5) Place a steamer rack inside the pot.
6) Put the jars on top of the rack.
7) Cover the pot.
8) Set it to manual.
9) Cook at high pressure for 5 minutes.
10) Release the pressure quickly.

Serving Suggestion: You can also set aside some cheese and use it for topping.
Tip: Use different colored bell peppers to make the dish colourful.
Nutritional Information Per Serving:

Calories   173
Total Fat 16g
Saturated Fat 8.4g
Cholesterol 184mg
Sodium 161mg
Total Carbohydrate 6.5g
Dietary Fiber 1.8g
Total Sugars 4.6g
Protein 11.1g
Potassium 356mg

9. COCONUT PORRIDGE

Serves: 6
Preparation time: 15 minutes
Ingredients:
1 cup dried coconut flakes
2 cups coconut milk
2 2/3 cups water
¼ cup coconut flour
¼ cup psyllium husks
1 teaspoon vanilla extract
½ teaspoon cinnamon
¼ teaspoon nutmeg
40 drops stevia liquid
Preparation:
1) Choose sauté setting.
2) Toast the coconut flakes until golden.
3) Add the water and coconut milk.
4) Secure the pot.
5) Select manual mode.
6) Cook at high pressure for 10 minutes.
7) Do a quick pressure release.
8) Stir in the rest of the ingredients before serving.

Serving Suggestion: Top the porridge with berry slices.
Tip: Use unsweetened coconut flakes.
Nutritional Information Per Serving:
Calories 303
Total Fat 25g
Saturated Fat 23g 1
Sodium 31mg
Potassium 242mg
Total Carbohydrates 17g
Dietary Fiber 11g
Sugars 1g
Protein 3g
Potassium 252 mg

10. Bacon Egg Bites

Serves: 8

Preparation time: 30 minutes

Ingredients:

4 eggs, beaten

¼ cup egg whites, beaten

¼ cup heavy whipping cream

½ cup cottage cheese

4 slices bacon, cooked and crumbled

½ red pepper, chopped

½ green pepper, chopped

1 cup red onion, chopped

1 cup shredded cheddar cheese

Salt and pepper to taste

Preparation:

1) Mix the eggs, egg whites, cream and cottage cheese.
2) Pour 1 cup of water into the Instant Pot.
3) Place a steamer rack inside the pot.
4) Pour the mixture into muffin tins.
5) Place the muffin tins on top of the rack.
6) Top each container with bacon, peppers and onion.
7) Cover the pot.
8) Set it to steam mode.
9) Release the pressure naturally.
10) Top with the cheddar cheese, and season with the salt and pepper before serving.

Serving Suggestion: Serve with low carb or keto crackers.

Tip: To prepare the dish faster, use a blender to mix the eggs, cheese and cream.

Nutritional Information Per Serving:

Calories   358

Total Fat 25.1g

Saturated Fat 12g

Cholesterol 227mg

Sodium 811mg

Total Carbohydrate 6.9g

Dietary Fiber 1.1g

Total Sugars 3g

Protein 25.9g

Potassium 348mg

11. Spicy Eggs & Kale

Serves: 2-4
Preparation time: 30 minutes
Ingredients:

1 tablespoon olive oil

½ onion, diced

2 cloves garlic, minced

½ red bell pepper, diced

½ teaspoon ground cumin

½ teaspoon smoked paprika

1 teaspoon chili powder

2 cups baby kale

1 ½ cups marinara sauce

½ teaspoon salt

½ teaspoon black pepper

4 eggs

Preparation:

1) Turn the Instant Pot to sauté setting.
2) Add the olive oil.
3) Cook the onion, garlic and bell pepper.
4) Season with the cumin, paprika and chili powder.
5) Add the kale.
6) Mix, and cook for 3 minutes.
7) Add the marinara sauce.
8) Sprinkle with the salt and pepper.
9) Let cool for 5 minutes.
10) Crack the eggs into the pot.
11) Cover the pot.
12) Cook at low pressure for 5 minutes.
13) Release the pressure quickly.

Serving Suggestion: Garnish with chopped parsley.

Tip: Cook a little longer if you want the eggs to be firm.

Nutritional Information Per Serving:

Calories   214

Total Fat 22.9g

Saturated Fat 8.6g

Cholesterol 166mg

Sodium 763mg

Total Carbohydrate 7.4g

Dietary Fiber 4.4g

Total Sugars 5.1g

Protein 9.3g

Potassium 436mg

12. Mushroom Quiche

Serves: 6
Preparation time: 20 minutes
Ingredients:
3 oz. Swiss cheese, shredded
2 oz. cremini mushrooms, chopped
1 scallion, chopped
4 eggs
¼ cup heavy cream
Salt to taste
Preparation:
1) Arrange the Swiss cheese in a silicon mold.
2) Place mushroom and scallion on top.
3) Mix the eggs, cream and salt in a blender.
4) Pour on top of the cheese and mushroom.
5) Pour 1 cup of water to the Instant Pot.
6) Place a steamer rack inside.
7) Put the silicone mold on top.
8) Close the pot.
9) Set it to manual.
10) Cook at high pressure for 5 minutes.
11) Let sit for 5 minutes before releasing the pressure naturally.
12) Flip the mold onto a serving plate.

Serving Suggestion: Garnish with chopped basil or parsley.

Tip: Use cream cheese if heavy cream is not available.

Nutritional Information Per Serving:
Calories   113
Total Fat 8.8g
Saturated Fat 4.3g
Cholesterol 129mg
Sodium 99mg
Total Carbohydrate 1.4g
Dietary Fiber 0.1g
Total Sugars 0.5g
Protein 8.1g
Potassium 92mg

13. Avocado & Egg Bites

Serves: 6
Preparation time: 25 minutes
Ingredients:

4 eggs
½ cup Mexican blend cheese
¼ cup heavy cream
½ cup cottage cheese
¼ teaspoon garlic powder
¼ teaspoon chili powder
¼ teaspoon cumin
Salt and pepper to taste
1 cup avocado, chopped

Preparation:

1) Pour 1 cup of water into the Instant Pot.
2) In a bowl, add all the ingredients except the avocado.
3) Pulse in the blender until smooth.
4) Pour the mixture into 4 silicone molds.
5) Place the mold on a steamer rack inside the pot.
6) Secure the lid.
7) Press the steam setting.
8) Set it to 10 minutes.
9) Release the pressure naturally.
10) Top with the chopped avocado.

Serving Suggestion: Sprinkle more cheese on top.

Tip: Skip the chilli powder if you don't like the dish to be spicy.

Nutritional Information Per Serving:

Calories 118
Total Fat 13g
Saturated Fat 6g
Cholesterol 115mg
Sodium 179mg
Total Carbohydrates 1g
Protein 7g
Potassium 101mg

14. Sausage & Veggies

Serves: 4
Preparation time: 30 minutes
Ingredients:

1 tablespoon olive oil

6 eggs

¼ cup almond milk

Salt and pepper to taste

6 oz. sausage, cooked

2 tablespoons onion, diced

¼ cup bell pepper, diced

¼ cup green onions, diced

2 tablespoons bacon bits

½ cup cheddar cheese, shredded

Preparation:

1) Coat a small baking dish with oil.
2) In a bowl, beat the eggs.
3) Whisk in the milk, salt and pepper.
4) Set the Instant Pot to sauté.
5) Brown the sausage for 3 minutes.
6) Pour the egg mixture into the baking dish.
7) Stir in the vegetables.
8) Top with the cooked sausage, bacon and cheese.
9) Cover the dish with foil.
10) Pour 2 cups of water into the pot.
11) Place a steamer rack inside.
12) Add the baking dish on top of the rack.
13) Cover the pot.
14) Set it to manual.
15) Cook at high pressure for 16 minutes.
16) Release the pressure naturally.
17) Let it cool, and then flip onto a plate.

Serving Suggestion: Top with more cheese.
Tip: Use both green and red bell pepper.
Nutritional Information Per Serving:

Calories 343

Total Fat 23g

Saturated Fat 9g

Cholesterol 293mg

Sodium 474mg

Total Carbohydrates 9g

Dietary Fiber 1g

Sugars 2g

Protein 20g

Potassium 329mg

15. TURKEY SAUSAGE, EGG & CHEESE

Serves: 6
Preparation time: 20 minutes
Ingredients:

12 eggs, beaten

1 cup almond milk

Salt and pepper to taste

3 cups turkey breakfast sausage

1 onion, diced

2 cups cheddar cheese, shredded

Preparation:

1) In a bowl, mix the eggs, almond milk, salt and pepper.
2) Coat the Instant Pot with cooking spray.
3) Pour the egg mixture into the pot.
4) Arrange a layer of the sausage, onion and cheese on top of the egg mixture.
5) Cover the pot.
6) Press the manual setting.
7) Cook at high pressure for 10 minutes.
8) Release the pressure naturally.

Serving Suggestion: Sprinkle chopped green onion on top.

Tip: Use ham or bacon in place of turkey sausage

Nutritional Information Per Serving:

Calories   377

Total Fat 30.8g

Saturated Fat 19.1g

Cholesterol 367mg

Sodium 364mg

Total Carbohydrate 5.1g

Dietary Fiber 1.3g

Total Sugars 3g

Protein 21.6g

Potassium 287mg

16. SAUSAGE CASSEROLE

Serves: 12
Preparation time: 30 minutes
Ingredients:

4 eggs, beaten

1 lb. breakfast sausage, cooked and drained

4 ½ tablespoons butter, melted

2 tablespoons sour cream

¼ teaspoon salt

2 cups Monterey Jack cheese, shredded

¼ cup coconut flour

¼ teaspoon baking powder

Preparation:

1) Coat a small baking dish with cooking spray.
2) In a bowl, combine all the ingredients. Mix well.
3) Pour the mixture into the baking dish.
4) Cover the dish with foil.
5) Place a steamer rack inside the Instant Pot.
6) Add the dish on top of the rack.
7) Pour 2 cups of water into the pot.
8) Cover the pot.
9) Set it to manual.
10) Cook at high pressure for 10 minutes.
11) Release the pressure naturally.

Serving Suggestion: Sprinkle more shredded cheese and chopped green onion on top.

Tip: You can also use cooked ham or bacon in place of the sausage.

Nutritional Information Per Serving:

Calories   262

Total Fat 22.6g

Saturated Fat 10.5g

Cholesterol 115mg

Sodium 487mg

Total Carbohydrate 0.4g

Dietary Fiber 0g

Total Sugars 0.2g

Protein 13.9g

Potassium 160mg

17. Egg Stuffed Avocado

Serves: 4
Preparation time: 20 minutes
Ingredients:
2 ripe avocados, sliced in half and pitted
4 eggs
Salt and pepper to taste
½ cup cheddar cheese, shredded
½ cup bacon, sliced into bits
Preparation:
1) Remove some of the flesh from the avocado to make room for the egg.
2) Place a steamer rack inside the Instant Pot.
3) Pour in 1 cup of water.
4) Add the avocados on top of the rack.
5) Crack an egg into each avocado slice.
6) Season with the salt and pepper.
7) Top with the cheese and bacon bits.
8) Cover the pot.
9) Set it to manual.
10) Cook at high pressure for 4 minutes.
11) Release the pressure quickly.

Serving Suggestion: Garnish with sliced chives.

Tip: You can also add more flavor by using herbs such as rosemary or thyme.

Nutritional Information Per Serving:
Calories   325
Total Fat 28.7g
Saturated Fat 9.5g
Cholesterol 179mg
Sodium 155mg
Total Carbohydrate 9.2g
Dietary Fiber 6.7g
Total Sugars 0.9g
Protein 11g
Potassium 561mg

18. Eggs with Herbs & Feta

Serves: 4
Preparation time: 10 minutes
Ingredients:

2 tablespoons butter, divided

1 teaspoon fresh thyme, chopped

2 tablespoons coconut milk, divided

4 eggs

1 tablespoon chives, chopped

2 tablespoons feta cheese, crumbled

Salt and pepper to taste

Preparation:

1) Brush a little butter on the bottoms and sides of 4 ramekins.
2) Add ½ tablespoons heavy cream into each of the ramekin.
3) Sprinkle each with thyme.
4) Crack 1 egg into each ramekin.
5) Top the eggs with chives.
6) Pour 1 cup of water into the Instant Pot.
7) Place a steamer rack inside the pot.
8) Add the ramekins on top of the rack.
9) Cover the pot.
10) Set it to manual.
11) Cook at high pressure for 2 minutes.
12) Release the pressure quickly.
13) Top with the feta cheese and season with salt and pepper.

Serving Suggestion: Garnish with chopped parsley.

Tip: You can also use half and half instead of coconut milk.

Nutritional Information Per Serving:

Calories   144

Total Fat 13g

Saturated Fat 7.3g

Cholesterol 183mg

Sodium 156mg

Total Carbohydrate 1.2g

Dietary Fiber 0.3g

Total Sugars 0.8g

Protein 6.5g

Potassium 88mg

19. Jalapeno Omelet

Serves: 6
Preparation time: 20 minutes
Ingredients:

Cooking spray
1 cup bacon, chopped
4 jalapeno pepper, seeded and chopped
12 eggs, beaten

¼ cup heavy cream
Salt and pepper to taste
1 cup cheddar cheese, shredded

Preparation:

1) Spray glass jars with oil.
2) Set the Instant Pot to sauté.
3) Cook the bacon until golden crisp.
4) Drain fat and set aside.
5) Add the jalapeno peppers to the pot.
6) Cook for 2 minutes.
7) In a bowl, whisk the eggs, cream, salt and pepper.
8) Fold in the peppers, bacon and cheese.
9) Pour the egg mixture into the glass jars.
10) Place a steamer rack inside the Instant Pot.
11) Pour in 2 cups of water.
12) Put the jars on top of the rack.
13) Cover the jars.
14) Cover the pot.
15) Set it to manual.
16) Cook at high pressure for 7 minutes.
17) Release the pressure naturally.

Serving Suggestion: Garnish top with chopped fresh herbs.

Tip: Cook only for 5 minutes if you want the eggs to be softer.

Nutritional Information Per Serving:

Calories   273
Total Fat 20.9g
Saturated Fat 9.2g
Cholesterol 364mg
Sodium 462mg

Total Carbohydrate 1.8g
Dietary Fiber 0.3g
Total Sugars 1.1g
Protein 19.5g
Potassium 214mg

20. CHEESY EGG BAKE

Serves: 4
Preparation time: 40 minutes
Ingredients:

6 slices bacon, chopped

1 cup spinach, chopped

6 eggs, beaten

¼ cup almond milk

½ cup cheddar cheese, shredded

Preparation:

1) Select the sauté function in the Instant Pot.
2) Cook the bacon until golden crisp.
3) Add the spinach.
4) Cook for 3 minutes.
5) In a bowl, whisk the eggs and the rest of the ingredients.
6) Pour the egg mixture into a small pan.
7) Fold in the spinach.
8) Top with the bacon.
9) Pour 2 cups of water into the Instant Pot.
10) Place a steamer rack inside the pot.
11) Put the baking dish on top of the rack.
12) Cover the pot.
13) Set it to manual.
14) Cook at high pressure for 20 minutes.
15) Release the pressure quickly.

Serving Suggestion: Top with more cheese and chopped red bell pepper.

Tip: Marinate the chicken longer for a more intense flavour but cover with foil and place inside the refrigerator.

Nutritional Information Per Serving:

Calories   342

Total Fat 26.8g

Saturated Fat 12.1g

Cholesterol 292mg

Sodium 847mg

Total Carbohydrate 2.2g

Dietary Fiber 0.5g

Total Sugars 1.1g

Protein 22.9g

Potassium 345mg

Chapter 12: 20 Keto Diet Meat Recipes

21. Pork Burrito Bowl

Serves: 4
Preparation time: 20 minutes
Ingredients:

1 ½ tablespoons pork lard
1 onion, sliced
2 bell peppers, sliced
1 clove garlic, chopped
Salt and pepper to taste

1 lb. pulled pork
½ cup chicken broth
6 cups lettuce, chopped
6 cups green cabbage, chopped
¼ cup guacamole

Preparation:

1) Choose the sauté setting in the Instant Pot.
2) Add the lard.
3) Wait for it to melt before adding the onion and bell pepper.
4) Cook for 2 minutes, stirring frequently.
5) Add the garlic, salt and pepper.
6) Stir well.
7) Add the pulled pork and chicken broth.
8) Cover the pot.
9) Set it to manual mode.
10) Cook at high pressure for 1 minute.
11) Release the pressure quickly.
12) Arrange the lettuce and green cabbage in serving bowls.
13) Add the pulled pork on top.
14) Top with the guacamole before serving.

Serving Suggestion: Additional options for toppings are salsa and sour cream.
Tip: You may also add ½ cup of water to avoid drying.
Nutritional Info:

Calories   417
Total Fat 95g
Saturated Fat 38.5g
Cholesterol 320mg
Sodium 2724mg

Total Carbohydrate 6g
Dietary Fiber 5.1g
Total Sugars 16.7g
Protein 75.6g
Potassium 476mg

22. MEXICAN BEEF

Serves: 6
Preparation time: 60 minutes
Ingredients:

2 ½ lb. beef brisket, sliced into cubes
Salt and pepper to taste
1 tablespoon chili powder
3 tablespoons ghee
1 tablespoon butter
1 onion, sliced

1 tablespoon tomato paste
6 cloves garlic, crushed
½ cup bone broth
½ teaspoon fish sauce
½ cup salsa

Preparation:

1) Season the beef with salt, pepper and chili powder.
2) Set the Instant Pot to sauté.
3) Add the ghee and butter.
4) Add the onion.
5) Cook until translucent.
6) Add the garlic and tomato paste.
7) Cook for 30 seconds.
8) Add the beef, bone broth, fish sauce and salsa.
9) Seal the pot.
10) Set it to manual.
11) Cook at high pressure for 35 minutes.
12) Release the pressure naturally.
13) Season with a little more salt and pepper before serving.

Serving Suggestion: Serve with chopped cilantro and sliced radish.
Tip: To decrease cooking time, you can slice the beef into smaller cubes.
Nutritional Info:

Calories   573
Total Fat 58.1g
Saturated Fat 23.9g
Cholesterol 731mg
Sodium 724mg

Total Carbohydrate 5.3g
Dietary Fiber 1.4g
Total Sugars 1.9g
Protein 42.2g
Potassium 3358mg

23. BEEF CURRY

Serves: 6
Preparation time: 60 minutes
Ingredients:
2.5 lb. beef stew chunks
3 zucchinis, chopped
1 lb. broccoli florets
½ cup chicken stock
1 tablespoon garlic power
2 tablespoons curry powder
Salt to taste
14 oz. coconut milk
1 tablespoon butter
Preparation:
1) Put all the ingredients except the coconut milk and butter in the Instant Pot.
2) Stir to combine.
3) Cover the pot.
4) Set it to manual.
5) Cook at high pressure for 45 minutes.
6) Release the pressure naturally.
7) Stir in the coconut milk and butter before serving.

Serving Suggestion: Serve with cauliflower rice.
Tip: You can also use other parts of beef such as beef brisket.
Nutritional Information:
Calories   485
Total Fat 50.1g
Saturated Fat 21.2g
Cholesterol 63mg
Sodium 1750mg
Total Carbohydrate 38.3g
Dietary Fiber 5.2g
Total Sugars 8.7g
Protein 20.2g
Potassium 704mg

24. BEEF SHORT RIBS

Serves: 4
Preparation time: 60 minutes
Ingredients:
2 lb. beef short ribs (boneless)
1 onion, chopped
3 tablespoons tamari sauce
2 tablespoons white wine
Salt and pepper to taste
Preparation:
1) Add the beef short ribs, onion, tamari sauce, white wine, salt and pepper in the Instant Pot.
2) Pour in 1 cup of water.
3) Mix well.
4) Seal the pot.
5) Press the stew button.
6) Set it to 45 minutes.
7) Release the pressure naturally.
Serving Suggestion: Serve with fresh green salad on the side.
Tip: Marinate the beef for 10 to 15 minutes before cooking. You can also add other spices such as curry powder and star anise.
Nutritional Info:
Calories   490
Total Fat 60.5g
Saturated Fat 10.8g
Cholesterol 206mg
Sodium 892mg
Total Carbohydrate 3.5g
Dietary Fiber 0.7g
Total Sugars 1.5g
Protein 47.2g
Potassium 900mg

25. POT ROAST WITH GRAVY

Serves: 6
Preparation time: 1 hour and 30 minutes
Ingredients:

Salt and pepper to taste

4 lb. chuck roast, sliced into 4 pieces

6 cloves garlic, peeled

4 sprigs thyme

1 sprig rosemary

2 parsnips, peeled

2 tablespoons balsamic vinegar

1 ½ cups beef broth

Preparation:

1) Rub the salt and pepper all over the chuck roast.
2) Place it in the Instant Pot.
3) Add the rest of the ingredients.
4) Mix well.
5) Secure the lid.
6) Choose manual mode.
7) Cook at high pressure for 60 minutes.
8) Release the pressure naturally.
9) Transfer the meat to a plate.
10) Shred with fork.
11) Transfer the contents of the Instant Pot to a blender.
12) Remove the herb sprigs.
13) Blend until smooth.
14) Season with the salt and pepper.
15) Pour the gravy on top of the beef before serving.

Serving Suggestion: Serve with mashed cauliflower. Top with chopped chives as garnish.

Tip: After seasoning the chuck roast, let sit for 5 to 10 minutes before cooking.

Nutritional Info:

Calories   704

Total Fat 55.7g

Saturated Fat 13.3g

Cholesterol 305mg

Sodium 396mg

Total Carbohydrate 9.8g

Dietary Fiber 2.6g

Total Sugars 2.4g

Protein 101.9g

Potassium 1115mg

26. PORK WITH CHIPOTLE CREAM SAUCE

Serves: 6
Preparation time: 1 hour and 30 minutes
Ingredients:

1 lb. pork tenderloin
Salt to taste
1 tablespoon garlic powder, divided
1 tablespoon chili powder, divided
1 tablespoon ground cumin, divided

1 tablespoon butter
14 ½ oz. canned tomatoes
¼ cup mayonnaise
3 tablespoons lime juice
1 ½ teaspoons chipotle powder

Preparation:

1) Season the pork tenderloin with the salt and half of the garlic powder, chili powder and cumin.
2) Press the sauté button in the Instant Pot.
3) Add the butter.
4) Add the pork tenderloin and cook for 4 minutes per side.
5) Pour in 4 cups of water.
6) Seal the pot.
7) Choose the stew setting.
8) Release the pressure naturally.
9) Transfer the pork to a bowl.
10) Shred with a fork.
11) Put the shredded fork back to the pot.
12) Add the remaining garlic powder, chilli powder and cumin.
13) Pour in the tomato sauce.
14) Simmer by pressing sauté.
15) Cook for 5 minutes.
16) While waiting, mix the mayo, lime juice and chipotle powder.
17) Top the pork with chipotle sauce before serving.

Serving Suggestion: Garnish with chopped cilantro.
Tip: You can use ghee or coconut oil instead of butter.
Nutritional Information:

Calories   290
Total Fat 32.4g
Saturated Fat 8.7g
Cholesterol 63mg
Sodium 172mg

Total Carbohydrate 7.8g
Dietary Fiber 1.5g
Total Sugars 3g
Protein 21.1g
Potassium 548mg

27. JAMAICAN PORK

Serves: 6
Preparation time: 60 minutes
Ingredients:
1 tablespoon olive oil
2 lb. pork shoulder
1/8 cup Jamaican Jerk spice blend
1 tablespoon butter
1/2 cup beef broth
Preparation:
1) Pour the olive oil all over the pork shoulder.
2) Sprinkle the spice blend on all sides.
3) Choose the sauté setting in the Instant Pot.
4) Add the butter to the pot.
5) Brown the beef on all sides.
6) Pour in the beef broth.
7) Cover the pot.
8) Set it to manual.
9) Cook at high pressure for 45 minutes.
10) Release the pressure naturally.
11) Shred the meat and top with the cooking liquid before serving.
Serving Suggestion: Garnish with chopped parsley.
Tip: You can also use beef stock or bone broth in place of the beef broth.
Nutritional Information:
Calories   482
Total Fat 56.7g
Saturated Fat 13.5g
Cholesterol 141mg
Sodium 180mg
Total Carbohydrate 0.1g
Dietary Fiber 0g
Total Sugars 0.1g
Protein 35.6g
Potassium 515mg

28. PORK WITH SAUERKRAUT

Serves: 6
Preparation time: 60 minutes
Ingredients:

3 lb. pork shoulder

Salt and pepper to taste

3 tablespoons butter

2 onion, chopped

3 cloves garlic, sliced

6 cups sauerkraut, divided

1 lb. hot dog, sliced and cooked

½ lb. kielbasa, sliced and cooked

Preparation:

1) Season the pork roast with salt and pepper.
2) Press the sauté setting in the Instant Pot.
3) Add the butter.
4) Brown the pork roast.
5) Pour in 2 cups of water, onion and garlic.
6) Season with a little more salt and pepper.
7) Seal the pot.
8) Set it to manual.
9) Cook at high pressure for 35 minutes.
10) Release the pressure naturally.
11) Shred the pork.
12) Stir in the sauerkraut, hotdog and kielbasa before serving.

Serving Suggestion: This dish goes well with any pickled vegetables.

Tip: You can also cook the hotdog and kielbasa in the Instant Pot using the sauté mode.

Nutritional Information:

Calories   792

Total Fat 83.5g

Saturated Fat 32.7g

Cholesterol 286mg

Sodium 851mg

Total Carbohydrate 14.6g

Dietary Fiber 5g

Total Sugars 6.7g

Protein 68.1g

Potassium 1167mg

29. Pork Chop with Mushrooms

Serves: 4
Preparation time: 60 minutes
Ingredients:

4 pork chops

2 tablespoons butter

2 tablespoons coconut oil, divided

1 cup chicken stock

1 onion sliced

8 oz. mushrooms, chopped

Salt and pepper to taste

Preparation:

1) Season the pork chops with the salt and pepper.
2) Add the butter and half of the coconut oil to the Instant Pot.
3) Set it to sauté.
4) Sear the pork chops for 2 minutes per side.
5) Remove from the pot and set aside.
6) Add the remaining coconut oil.
7) Add the onion and cook for 2 minutes.
8) Add the mushrooms and cook for another 2 minutes.
9) Pour in the chicken stock.
10) Scrape the brown bits using a wooden spoon.
11) Put the pork chops back to the pot.
12) Seal the pot.
13) Set it to manual.
14) Cook at high pressure for 10 minutes.
15) Release the pressure quickly.
16) Remove the pork chops.
17) Press sauté.
18) Add the remaining coconut oil. Cook for 5 minutes.
19) Pour cooking liquid on top of the pork chops before serving.

Serving Suggestion: Serve with fresh green salad.

Tip: Add a sprinkle of dried basil to the pork chops.

Nutritional Information:

Calories   391

Total Fat 32.8g

Saturated Fat 17g

Cholesterol 84mg

Sodium 292mg

Total Carbohydrate 4.6g

Dietary Fiber 1.2g

Total Sugars 2.3g

Protein 20.3g

Potassium 501mg

30. Spiced Pork Chops

Serves: 4
Preparation time: 45 minutes
Ingredients:

4 pork chops
1 teaspoon onion powder
1 teaspoon garlic powder
1 teaspoon cayenne pepper
Salt and pepper to taste

2 tablespoons coconut oil
1 tablespoon butter
6 oz. mushrooms
½ cup heavy cream

Preparation:

1) In a bowl, combine the onion powder, garlic powder, cayenne pepper, salt and pepper.
2) Season the pork chops with 1 tablespoon of this mixture.
3) Set the Instant Pot to sauté.
4) Brown the pork chops for 3 minutes per side.
5) Transfer the pork chops to a plate.
6) Add the onions and mushrooms in the Instant Pot.
7) Put the pork chops on top.
8) Close the pot.
9) Set it to manual.
10) Cook at high pressure for 25 minutes.
11) Release the pressure naturally.
12) Transfer the pork chops, mushrooms and onions on a serving platter.
13) Mix the remaining spices, heavy cream and butter in the pot.
14) Press sauté and simmer for 5 minutes.
15) Pour the gravy on top of the pork chops before serving.

Serving Suggestion: Serve with any vegetable dish or green salad.

Tip: After seasoning the pork chops, let sit for a few minutes before cooking.

Nutritional Information:

Calories   407
Total Fat 55.3g
Saturated Fat 22.6g
Cholesterol 97mg
Sodium 85mg

Total Carbohydrate 3.1g
Dietary Fiber 0.7g
Total Sugars 1.2g
Protein 19.9g
Potassium 445mg

31. CHORIZO CHILI

Serves: 6
Preparation time: 40 minutes
Ingredients:

1 ½ tablespoons olive oil

1 onion, chopped

1 celery stick, cubed

7 oz. chorizo sausage, diced

½ carrot, cubed

1 red chili, diced

3 cloves garlic, diced

2.2 lb. ground beef

3 teaspoons cumin

2 cups canned tomatoes

4 tablespoon tomato paste

1 tablespoon soy sauce

2 bay leaves

Salt to taste

Preparation:

1) Set the Instant Pot to sauté.
2) Add the olive oil.
3) Cook the onion, celery, chorizo, carrot and chilli for 4-5 minutes.
4) Add the garlic, beef and the rest of the ingredients.
5) Mix well.
6) Secure the lid.
7) Press manual mode.
8) Cook at high pressure for 15 minutes.
9) Release the pressure naturally.
10) Season with the salt.

Serving Suggestion: Serve with chopped avocado on the side.

Tip: Add chili powder if you like your dish spicy.

Nutritional Information:

Calories   568

Total Fat 43g

Saturated Fat 12.8g

Cholesterol 176mg

Sodium 554mg

Total Carbohydrate 7.7g

Dietary Fiber 1.8g

Total Sugars 4g

Protein 58.6g

Potassium 1091mg

32. Pork & Cauliflower Gravy

Serves: 5
Preparation time: 1 hour and 20 minutes
Ingredients:

1 onion, chopped
4 cloves garlic, crushed and minced
4 cups cauliflower, chopped
2 ribs celery
3 lb. pork roast

Salt and pepper to taste
8 oz. mushrooms, sliced
2 tablespoons coconut oil
2 tablespoons ghee

Preparation:

1) Add the onion, garlic, cauliflower and celery in the Instant Pot.
2) Put the pork roast on top.
3) Season the pork roast with salt and pepper.
4) Pour in 2 cups of water.
5) Cover the pot.
6) Set it to manual.
7) Cook at high pressure for 60 minutes.
8) Release the pressure quickly.
9) Transfer the pork roast to a baking pan.
10) Bake in the oven at 400 degrees F for 5 minutes.
11) Meanwhile, prepare the gravy transferring the pot contents to a blender.
12) Blend until smooth.
13) Press sauté in the Instant Pot.
14) Pour in the coconut oil and ghee.
15) Add the mushrooms and the blended mixture.
16) Cook for 5 minutes.
17) Serve the pot roast with the mushrooms and gravy.

Serving Suggestion: A bowl of fresh green salad or steamed vegetables goes well with this dish.

Tip: If the pot roast is frozen, cook at high pressure for 90 minutes.

Nutritional Information:

Calories   697
Total Fat 56.4g
Saturated Fat 27.2g
Cholesterol 247mg
Sodium 180mg

Total Carbohydrate 8.6g
Dietary Fiber 3g
Total Sugars 3.7g
Protein 81g
Potassium 1523mg

33. TOMATO MEATBALLS

Serves: 4
Preparation time: 30 minutes
Ingredients:

1.3 lb. ground beef

1 teaspoon garlic powder

1 teaspoon onion powder

1 teaspoon dried oregano

Salt to taste

2 tablespoons olive oil

1 onion, diced

2 cloves garlic, diced

2 cups canned tomatoes

Preparation:

1) Mix the ground beef, garlic powder, onion powder, oregano and salt in a bowl.
2) Form 8-10 meatballs.
3) Choose the sauté function in the Instant Pot.
4) Add the olive oil, onion and garlic.
5) Cook for 5 minutes, stirring frequently.
6) Add the meatballs.
7) Pour in the tomato sauce.
8) Mix well.
9) Lock the lid in place.
10) Press manual.
11) Cook at high pressure for 5 minutes.
12) Release the pressure naturally.

Serving Suggestion: Serve with cauliflower rice or spaghetti squash.

Tip: Add chili powder if you like your meatballs spicy.

Nutritional Information:

Calories   369

Total Fat 26.5g

Saturated Fat 7.5g

Cholesterol 132mg

Sodium 142mg

Total Carbohydrate 7.8g

Dietary Fiber 2g

Total Sugars 4g

Protein 46.1g

Potassium 873mg

34. Corned Beef with Cabbage

Serves: 12
Preparation time: 1 hour and 45 minutes
Ingredients:

4 lb. corned beef brisket

2 teaspoons black peppercorns

2 teaspoon dried mustard

4 cloves garlic, crushed

2 onions, sliced

8 cups cabbage, chopped

Preparation:

1) Place the corned beef in the Instant Pot.
2) Add 6 cups of water.
3) Add the peppercorns, dried mustard and garlic.
4) Mix well.
5) Cover the pot.
6) Set it to stew setting.
7) Release the pressure naturally.
8) Transfer the beef brisket to a plate.
9) Add the onion and cabbage to the pot.
10) Close the pot.
11) Choose the soup function.
12) Cook for 15 minutes.
13) Release the pressure quickly.
14) Put back the beef to the pot.
15) Press sauté and simmer for 5 minutes.

Serving Suggestion: Sprinkle with a little salt before serving.
Tip: Add chopped celery stalks to the dish for extra flavor.
Nutritional Information:

Calories 334

Total Fat 32.8g

Saturated Fat 7.2g

Cholesterol 81mg

Sodium 1882mg

Total Carbohydrates 8.1g

Dietary Fiber 2.6g

Sugars 3.7g

Protein 23.7g

35. Beef Roast

Serves: 6
Preparation time: 1 hour and 20 minutes
Ingredients:

2 tablespoons olive oil

1 tablespoon butter

4 lb. beef chuck roast

16 oz. jarred pepperoncini peppers, sliced

½ onion, sliced thinly

2 cloves garlic, crushed and minced

1 cup beef broth

1 tablespoon onion powder

1 tablespoon oregano

1 tablespoon parsley

1 teaspoon basil

1 tablespoon garlic salt

Salt and pepper to taste

Preparation:

1) Press the sauté function in the Instant Pot.
2) Add the olive oil and butter.
3) Brown the beef on all sides for 4-6 minutes.
4) Add half of the pepperoncini peppers.
5) Pour in ¼ cup of its juice.
6) Add the onion, garlic, beef broth and the rest of the ingredients.
7) Seal the pot.
8) Set it to manual.
9) Cook at high pressure for 70 minutes.
10) Release the pressure naturally.
11) Shred the meat before serving.
12) Top with the remaining pepperoncini.

Serving Suggestion: Enjoy this dish with buttered corn.

Tip: To save time, you can replace the seasonings with a dry seasoning pack of Italian dressing.

Nutritional Information:

Calories   1177

Total Fat 91.1g

Saturated Fat 35.5g

Cholesterol 317mg

Sodium 336mg

Total Carbohydrate 3.8g

Dietary Fiber 0.8g

Total Sugars 1.3g

Protein 80.6g

Potassium 785mg

36. MEATBALLS IN CREAM SAUCE

Serves: 6
Preparation time: 35 minutes
Ingredients:

1 ¼ lb. ground pork

½ onion, minced

1 clove garlic, crushed and minced

1 egg, beaten

2 strips bacon, minced

2 tablespoons almond flour

Salt and pepper to taste

1 tablespoon soy sauce

1 tablespoon tomato paste

2 tablespoons avocado oil

1 ½ cups chicken stock

2 tablespoons butter, melted

2/3 cup heavy cream

Preparation:

1) Combine the ground pork, onion, garlic, egg, bacon, almond flour, salt, pepper and soy sauce in a bowl.
2) Form 12 meatballs from the mixture.
3) Choose the sauté function in the Instant Pot.
4) Add the avocado oil.
5) Cook the meatballs until brown.
6) Transfer to a plate and set aside.
7) Pour the chicken stock into the pot.
8) Scrape the brown bits with a wooden spoon.
9) Put the meatballs back to the pot.
10) Cover the pot.
11) Set it to manual.
12) Cook at high pressure for 7 minutes.
13) Release the pressure naturally.
14) Stir in the butter, cream and a little more salt and pepper.
15) Press sauté to simmer for 2 minutes.

Serving Suggestion: Serve on top of spaghetti squash.

Tip: If avocado oil is not available, you can use coconut oil instead.

Nutritional Information:

Calories   446

Total Fat 30.7g

Saturated Fat 9.3g

Cholesterol 214mg

Sodium 652mg

Total Carbohydrate 3g

Dietary Fiber 0.7g

Total Sugars 1.1g

Protein 58.9g

Potassium 999mg

37. SWEET & SPICY PORK

Serves: 6
Preparation time: 2 hours
Ingredients:

1 cup bone broth

4 lb. pork shoulder

6 cloves garlic, crushed and minced

½ cup coconut aminos

3 tablespoons lard

¼ cup Keto sweetener

2 tablespoons rice wine vinegar

1 teaspoon dried ginger

1 tablespoon Chinese five-spice

1 teaspoon turmeric

½ tablespoon lime juice

1 teaspoon lime zest

Preparation:

1) Choose the sauté function in the Instant Pot.
2) Pour in the bone broth.
3) Add the pork roast.
4) Mix the rest of the ingredients in a bowl.
5) Pour the mixture over the pork roast.
6) Cover the pot.
7) Set it to manual.
8) Cook at high pressure for 90 minutes.
9) Release the pressure naturally.
10) Remove the pork shoulder from the pot.
11) Shred with a fork.
12) Put it back to the pot.
13) Press sauté and simmer until sauce is reduced to half.

Serving Suggestion: Stuff the pork shreds in low carb tacos.

Tip: If you like it spicy, add a teaspoon or more of sriracha sauce.

Nutritional Information:

Calories   959

Total Fat 71.2g

Saturated Fat 26.3g

Cholesterol 278mg

Sodium 216mg

Total Carbohydrate 2.8g

Dietary Fiber 0.2g

Total Sugars 0.1g

Protein 71g

Potassium 1025mg

38. Taco Meat

Serves: 8
Preparation time: 15 minutes
Ingredients:
1 teaspoon olive oil
1 teaspoon butter
2 lb. ground beef
½ cup onion, diced
½ cup bell pepper, diced
1 cup tomato sauce
3 tablespoons taco seasoning
Preparation:
1) Choose the sauté function in the Instant Pot.
2) Add the olive oil and butter to the pot. Mix.
3) Brown the ground beef.
4) Add the rest of the ingredients. Mix well.
5) Cover the pot.
6) Set it to manual.
7) Cook at high pressure for 8 minutes.
8) Release the pressure quickly.

Serving Suggestion: Garnish with fresh cilantro.
Tip: You can also use minced beef in place of ground beef.
Nutritional Information:
Calories 194
Total Fat 10g
Saturated Fat 2g
Cholesterol 83mg
Sodium 88mg
Total Carbohydrates 4g
Sugars 2g
Protein 21g
Potassium 419mg

39. BUTTER BEEF

Serves: 6
Preparation time: 1 hour and 15 minutes
Ingredients:
3 lb. beef roast
1 tablespoon olive oil
2 tablespoons ranch dressing seasoning mix
2 tablespoons zesty Italian seasoning mix
1 jar pepper rings
1 stick butter
Preparation:
1) Set the Instant Pot to sauté.
2) Add the olive oil into the pot.
3) Sear the beef roast on all sides.
4) Pour in 4 cups of water.
5) Add the seasonings and pepper rings.
6) Place butter stick on top of the roast.
7) Seal the pot.
8) Set it to manual.
9) Cook at high pressure for 60 minutes.
10) Release the pressure naturally.
11) Slice the beef before serving.

Serving Suggestion: Serve with pureed cauliflower.
Tip: You can also shred the beef using 2 forks.
Nutritional Information:
Calories   582
Total Fat 31.7g
Saturated Fat 15.3g
Cholesterol 243mg
Sodium 402mg
Total Carbohydrate 1.1g
Dietary Fiber 0g
Total Sugars 0.1g
Protein 69g
Potassium 918mg

40. BEEF & BROCCOLI

Serves: 4
Preparation time: 60 minutes
Ingredients:
2 lb. flank steak, sliced
2/3 cup liquid aminos
1 cup beef stock
3 tablespoons alternative sweetener
3 garlic cloves, crushed and minced
1 teaspoon ginger, grated
½ teaspoon red pepper flakes
Salt to taste
2 cups broccoli, sliced into florets
1 red bell pepper, sliced
Preparation:
1) Add the steak, liquid aminos, beef stock, sweetener, garlic, ginger, red pepper and salt in the Instant Pot.
2) Seal the pot.
3) Select manual mode.
4) Cook at high pressure for 30 minutes.
5) Release the pressure naturally.
6) Stir in the vegetables into the pot.
7) Press sauté and cook for 20 minutes before serving.

Serving Suggestion: Sprinkle with sesame seeds before serving.
Tip: You can use soy sauce or tamari in place of liquid aminos.
Nutritional Information:
Calories   475
Total Fat 19.3g
Saturated Fat 7.9g
Cholesterol 125mg
Sodium 378mg
Total Carbohydrate 6.5g
Dietary Fiber 1.8g
Total Sugars 2.3g
Protein 65.6g
Potassium 1019mg

CHAPTER 13: 20 KETO DIET CHICKEN & POULTRY RECIPES

41. CHICKEN IN TOMATO WALNUT SAUCE

Serves: 6
Preparation time: 2 hours and 45 minutes
Ingredients:

4 lb. chicken

½ cup avocado oil, divided

1 ½ tablespoons sun-dried tomatoes, chopped

8 cloves garlic, minced

1 onion, chopped

2 teaspoons Italian seasoning

¼ cup walnuts, chopped

1 tablespoon lemon juice

1 cup bone broth

Preparation:

1) Pour 1/3 cup of avocado oil in a blender.
2) Add the tomatoes, garlic, onion and Italian seasoning. Pulse until smooth.
3) Gradually add the walnuts. Keep blending until well combined.
4) Coat the chicken with lemon juice. Let it sit for 5 minutes.
5) Soak the chicken in the walnut mixture. Marinate for 2 hours.
6) Set the Instant Pot to sauté. Pour in the remaining avocado oil.
7) Brown the chicken for 3 minutes per side. Pour in the bone broth.
8) Give it a good mix.
9) Cover the pot.
10) Set it to manual.
11) Cook at high pressure for 25 minutes.
12) Release the pressure naturally.

Serving Suggestion: Garnish with lemon wedges before serving.

Tip: Use freshly squeezed lemon juice.

Nutritional Information:

Calories 532

Total Fat 35.1g

Saturated Fat 7.3g

Cholesterol 234mg

Sodium 193mg

Total Carbohydrate 4.9g

Dietary Fiber 1.7g

Total Sugars 1.2g

Protein 89.6g

Potassium 702mg

42. FRENCH GARLIC CHICKEN

Serves: 4
Preparation time: 50 minutes
Ingredients:

2 tablespoons olive oil

1 tablespoon cider vinegar

2 teaspoons herbes de Provence

Salt and pepper to taste

Garlic powder to taste

1 tablespoon Dijon mustard

1 lb. chicken thighs (boneless and skinless)

2 tablespoons butter

8 cloves garlic, chopped

¼ cup water

¼ cup cream

Preparation:

1) Combine the olive oil, vinegar, herbes de Provence, salt, pepper and garlic powder in a bowl.
2) Marinate the chicken thighs in half of the mixture for 30 minutes. Reserve the other half.
3) Set the Instant Pot to sauté.
4) Add the butter.
5) Once melted, add the garlic.
6) Cook for 3 minutes.
7) Add the chicken and cook for 3-5 minutes per side.
8) Add the reserved marinade and water.
9) Seal the pot. Set it to manual.
10) Cook at high pressure for 10 minutes.
11) Release the pressure naturally.
12) Transfer the chicken to a serving platter.
13) Stir the cream into the pot.
14) Pour the sauce over the chicken.

Serving Suggestion: Garnish with chopped parsley.

Tip: You can also try topping the chicken with a little Parmesan.

Nutritional Information:

Calories 349

Total Fat 32.2g

Saturated Fat 7.5g

Cholesterol 119mg

Sodium 189mg

Total Carbohydrate 2.8g

Dietary Fiber 0.3g

Total Sugars 0.4g

Protein 33.6g

Potassium 316mg

43. Chicken Toscana

Serves: 6
Preparation time: 1 hour and 10 minutes
Ingredients:

Salt and pepper to taste

3 lb. chicken thighs

1 teaspoon dried rosemary

2 tablespoons olive oil

1 cup dry white wine

2 zucchinis, sliced

6 oz. Kalamata olives, sliced in half

8 oz. mushrooms

6 oz. roasted red peppers

6 oz. jarred artichoke hearts

Preparation:

1) Rub the salt and pepper all over the chicken.
2) Season it with the dried rosemary.
3) Choose the sauté function in the Instant Pot.
4) Pour in the olive oil.
5) Brown the chicken for 5 minutes per side.
6) Pour in the white wine.
7) Seal the pot.
8) Select poultry mode.
9) Release the pressure quickly.
10) Add the rest of the ingredients.
11) Cover the pot.
12) Select manual setting.
13) Cook at high pressure for 1 minute.
14) Release the pressure quickly.

Serving Suggestion: Sprinkle with chopped fresh basil and fresh parsley before serving.
Tip: Chicken breasts can also be used for this recipe.
Nutritional Information:

Calories   569

Total Fat 34.8g

Saturated Fat 7.7g

Cholesterol 202mg

Sodium 608mg

Total Carbohydrate 9.7g

Dietary Fiber 2.9g

Total Sugars 3.8g

Protein 68.4g

Potassium 933mg

44. Chicken in Garlic Butter Sauce

Serves: 4
Preparation time: 50 minutes
Ingredients:
4 chicken breasts, sliced
¼ cup ghee mixed with 1 teaspoon turmeric powder
Salt to taste
10 cloves garlic, diced
3 tablespoons butter
Preparation:

1) Place the chicken breasts inside the Instant Pot.
2) Add the ghee and turmeric mixture, salt and garlic.
3) Cover the pot.
4) Set it to manual.
5) Cook at high pressure for 35 minutes.
6) Release the pressure naturally.
7) Mix in the butter before serving.

Serving Suggestion: Sprinkle dried basil before serving.
Tip: You can also cook the chicken breast whole, and then shred with a fork afterwards.
Nutritional Information:
Calories   200
Total Fat 31.4g
Saturated Fat 13.4g
Cholesterol 56mg
Sodium 102mg
Total Carbohydrate 2.5g
Dietary Fiber 0.2g
Total Sugars 0.1g
Protein 0.7g
Potassium 33mg

45. CHICKEN & MUSHROOM

Serves: 4
Preparation time: 30 minutes
Ingredients:

2 tablespoons butter
6 cloves garlic, sliced
1 cup onion, sliced
2 cups mushrooms
1 lb. chicken thighs
1 teaspoon dried thyme

Salt and pepper to taste
2 tablespoons water
4 cups baby spinach
½ cup heavy whipping cream
½ tablespoon lemon juice

Preparation:

1) Set the Instant Pot to sauté.
2) Add the butter.
3) Cook the garlic for 1 minute.
4) Add the onion and mushroom.
5) Cook for 3 minutes.
6) Add the rest of the ingredients, placing the spinach on top.
7) Cover the pot.
8) Set it to manual.
9) Cook at high pressure for 8 minutes.
10) Release the pressure naturally.
11) Press sauté.
12) Stir in the cream and lemon juice.

Serving Suggestion: Garnish with lemon slices.
Tip: Use freshly squeezed lemon juice.
Nutritional Information:

Calories   352
Total Fat 20g
Saturated Fat 9.5g
Cholesterol 137mg
Sodium 172mg
Total Carbohydrate 7.1g
Dietary Fiber 1.8g
Total Sugars 2.1g
Protein 35.8g
Potassium 632mg

46. CHICKEN WITH BACON & CHEESE

Serves: 4
Preparation time: 40 minutes
Ingredients:

6 strips bacon

4 chicken breasts

2 tablespoons butter

½ teaspoon thyme

½ teaspoon garlic salt

¾ cup chicken stock

¼ cup heavy whipping cream

2 oz. cream cheese

Salt and pepper to taste

Preparation:

1) Choose the sauté setting in the Instant Pot.
2) Cook the bacon until golden crisp.
3) Take half of the bacon, chop and set aside.
4) Add the chicken breasts to the pot.
5) Add the butter, thyme, garlic salt, and chicken stock.
6) Cover the pot.
7) Set it to manual.
8) Cook at high pressure for 11 minutes.
9) Release the pressure naturally.
10) Take the chicken out and shred using 2 forks.
11) Put the shredded chicken back to the pot.
12) Press the sauté function.
13) Stir in the whipping cream and cream cheese.
14) Season with the salt and pepper.

Serving Suggestion: Sprinkle with the crumbled bacon bits and cheddar cheese or parmesan before serving.

Tip: If you'd like the sauce to be thicker, you can add xanthan gum.

Nutritional Information:

Calories   648

Total Fat 44g

Saturated Fat 17.4g

Cholesterol 191mg

Sodium 1272mg

Total Carbohydrate 9.1g

Dietary Fiber 0.5g

Total Sugars 0.3g

Protein 46.8g

Potassium 475mg

47. CRACK CHICKEN

Serves: 6
Preparation time: 20 minutes
Ingredients:
1 cup bone broth
2 lb. chicken tenders
Salt and pepper to taste
12 oz. cream cheese
8 oz. bacon, cooked and crumbled
½ cup cheddar cheese
Preparation:
1) Pour the bone broth into the Instant Pot.
2) Season the chicken with the salt and pepper.
3) Add the chicken and cream cheese into the pot.
4) Cover the pot.
5) Set it to manual.
6) Cook at high pressure for 10 minutes.
7) Release the pressure naturally.
8) Stir in the bacon and cheddar cheese.
9) Cover the pot and wait for the cheese to melt before serving.

Serving Suggestion: Serve with any low carb grilled vegetables.

Tip: If you're going to use chicken breasts, increase cooking time to 12 minutes.
Nutritional Information:
Calories   440
Total Fat 38.4g
Saturated Fat 8g
Cholesterol 181.3mg
Sodium 396.7mg
Total Carbohydrate 3.5g
Dietary Fiber 0g
Sugars 2.2g
Protein 41.1g

48. SPICY WINGS

Serves: 4
Preparation time: 2 hours and 15 minutes
Ingredients:

Salt and pepper to taste
2 lb. chicken wings
1 cup hot sauce
3 cloves garlic, crushed and minced
3 tablespoons lime juice
1 tablespoons avocado oil
1 cup sour cream
½ cup parsley, chopped
3 chives, chopped
1 teaspoon dried dill
½ teaspoon cayenne pepper
1 teaspoon paprika

Preparation:

1) Rub the salt and pepper all over the chicken.
2) Pour half of the hot sauce over the chicken.
3) Marinate for 2 hours.
4) Set the Instant Pot to sauté.
5) Add the avocado oil.
6) Brown the wings for 2-3 minutes per side.
7) Add the lime juice, remaining hot sauce, garlic and lime juice to the pot.
8) Secure the lid.
9) Set it to manual.
10) Cook at high pressure for 5 minutes.
11) Release the pressure quickly.
12) In a bowl, combine the rest of the ingredients.
13) Serve the chicken with the ranch dressing.

Serving Suggestion: Serve with zucchini sticks or cucumber rounds.

Tip: You can also add minced garlic to the ranch dressing.

Nutritional Information Per Serving:

Calories   577
Total Fat 39.7g
Saturated Fat 16.3g
Cholesterol 227mg
Sodium 1754mg
Total Carbohydrate 6.4g
Dietary Fiber 1g
Total Sugars 1.2g
Protein 68.3g
Potassium 817mg

49. CHICKEN TACO

Serves: 8
Preparation time: 55 minutes
Ingredients:

4 chicken breasts, sliced into strips

1 teaspoon garlic powder

1 teaspoon onion powder

½ cup salsa

1 tablespoon hot sauce

4 oz. cream cheese

2 tablespoons lime juice

4 oz. green chili, diced

¾ cup Mexican blend cheese, grated

8 low-carb tortillas

Preparation:

1) Put the chicken strips inside the Instant Pot.
2) Add the garlic powder, onion powder and salsa.
3) Secure the lid.
4) Set it to manual.
5) Cook at high pressure for 8 minutes.
6) Release the pressure naturally.
7) Take the chicken strips and shred with 2 forks.
8) Add shredded chicken back to the pot.
9) Add the hot sauce, cream cheese, lime juice, green chilli and cheese blend. Stir and let sit for 1 minute.
10) While waiting, heat the tortillas in a pan.
11) Stuff each tortilla with the chicken mixture.

Serving Suggestion: Additional options for toppings include sliced olives, chopped chives, sour cream and avocado cubes.

Tip: You can also use the same recipe for nachos.

Nutritional Information:

Calories   492

Total Fat 28.2g

Saturated Fat 13.9g

Cholesterol 187mg

Sodium 893mg

Total Carbohydrate 6.9g

Dietary Fiber 0.6g

Total Sugars 3.6g

Protein 50.4g

Potassium 525mg

50. WHOLE CHICKEN

Serves: 6-8
Preparation time: 50 minutes
Ingredients:
1 whole chicken
Garlic salt to taste
Pepper to taste
3 teaspoons dried rosemary
3 tablespoons coconut oil
Preparation:
1) Pour 1 cup of water into the Instant Pot.
2) Place a steamer rack inside.
3) Coat the chicken with garlic salt, pepper and rosemary.
4) Put the chicken on top of the steamer rack.
5) Cover the pot.
6) Set it to manual.
7) Cook at high pressure for 20 minutes.
8) Release the pressure naturally.
Serving Suggestion: Serve with grilled vegetables.
Tip: Let the chicken cool for 1 to 2 minutes before slicing and serving.
Nutritional Information Per Serving:
Calories   429
Total Fat 21.2g
Saturated Fat 9.9g
Cholesterol 173mg
Sodium 169mg
Total Carbohydrate 0.1g
Dietary Fiber 0g
Total Sugars 0g
Protein 56.3g
Potassium 474mg

51. Belizean Chicken

Serves: 4
Preparation time: 1 hour and 25 minutes
Ingredients:

2 tablespoons achiote seasoning

3 tablespoons Worcestershire sauce

Black pepper to taste

1 teaspoon dried oregano

1 teaspoon ground cumin

2 tablespoons white vinegar

1 teaspoon alternative sweetener

4 chicken legs

1 tablespoon coconut oil

1 cup onion, sliced

3 cloves garlic, sliced

2 cups chicken stock

Preparation:

1) In a bowl, mix the achiote paste, Worcestershire sauce, pepper, oregano, cumin, vinegar and sweetener.
2) Marinate the chicken in half of this mixture for 1 hour. Reserve the remaining marinade.
3) Set the Instant Pot to sauté.
4) Pour in the coconut oil.
5) Brown the chicken for 2 minutes per side.
6) Remove the chicken from the pot and set aside.
7) Add the onion and garlic.
8) Cook for 2 minutes.
9) Put the chicken back.
10) Add the chicken stock.
11) Secure the pot.
12) Set it to manual.
13) Cook at high pressure for 20 minutes.
14) Release the pressure naturally.
15) Stir in the remaining marinade.
16) Press sauté and simmer the sauce for 2-3 minutes.

Serving Suggestion: Serve with ketchup and mayonnaise.
Tip: For a more intense flavor, add more herbs such as oregano and basil.

52. RANCH CHICKEN

Serves: 8
Preparation time: 60 minutes
Ingredients:
1 tablespoon olive oil
1 tablespoon red wine vinegar
2 tablespoons taco seasoning
2 tablespoons ranch seasoning
¾ cup low sodium chicken broth
2 lb. chicken breasts
Preparation:
1) In a bowl, mix the olive oil, red wine vinegar, taco seasoning, ranch seasoning and chicken broth.
2) Marinate the chicken in the mixture for 30 minutes.
3) Add the chicken and marinade to the Instant Pot.
4) Cover the pot.
5) Set it to poultry.
6) Release the pressure naturally.
7) Shred the chicken before serving.
Serving Suggestion: Serve on lettuce cups.
Tip: If you want to use manual setting, cook at high pressure for 15 minutes.
Nutritional Information:
Calories 148
Total Fat 12g
Saturated Fat 6g
Cholesterol 72mg
Sodium 138mg
Potassium 438mg
Protein 24g

53. LEMON GARLIC CHICKEN

Serves: 4
Preparation time: 30 minutes
Ingredients:

8 chicken thighs (boneless)

Salt and pepper to taste

½ teaspoon smoked paprika

½ teaspoon garlic powder

2 tablespoons olive oil

3 tablespoons butter

½ onion, chopped

6 garlic cloves, minced

1 tablespoon lemon juice

1 ½ tablespoons Italian seasoning

¼ cup chicken broth

1 teaspoon lemon zest

2 tablespoons heavy cream

Preparation:

1) Rub the chicken with salt, pepper, paprika and garlic powder.
2) Set the Instant Pot to sauté.
3) Pour in the olive oil.
4) Brown the chicken for 3 minutes per side.
5) Add the butter to the pot. Add the onions and garlic. Cook for 1 minute.
6) Deglaze the pot by pouring lemon juice
7) Add the Italian seasoning, chicken broth and lemon zest.
8) Mix well. Seal the pot. Choose manual mode.
9) Cook at high pressure for 7 minutes.
10) Release the pressure naturally. Remove the chicken from the pot.
11) Stir in the cream to the cooking liquid.
12) Press sauté and let the sauce cook until thick.
13) Pour the sauce over the chicken before serving.

Serving Suggestion: Garnish with lemon wedges and chopped parsley.

Tip: Use arrowroot powder if you want the sauce to be thicker.

Nutritional Information Per Serving:

Calories 558

Total Fat 46g

Saturated Fat 15g

Cholesterol 198mg

Sodium 268mg

Total Carbohydrates 6g

Dietary Fiber 1g

Sugars 1g

Protein 28g

Potassium 435mg

54. TURKEY & VEGGIES

Serves: 6
Preparation time: 20 minutes
Ingredients:

1 tablespoon olive oil
1 tablespoon butter
1 lb. ground turkey
1 ½ tablespoons chili paste
1 onion, chopped
2 teaspoons garlic, minced

1 ½ cups bell pepper, chopped
1 cup zucchini, chopped
1 cup vegetable broth
1 cup tomato sauce
14 oz. canned tomatoes

Preparation:

1) Choose the sauté setting in the Instant Pot.
2) Pour in the olive oil.
3) Add the ground turkey.
4) Cook until brown.
5) Add the rest of the ingredients.
6) Mix well.
7) Secure the lid.
8) Set it to manual.
9) Cook at high pressure for 8 minutes.
10) Do a quick pressure release.

Serving Suggestion: Enjoy this dish with a cup of cauliflower rice.

Tip: Try using fire-roasted tomatoes for a more intense flavor.

Nutritional Information Per Serving:

Calories 156
Total Fat 12g
Saturated fat 7g
Cholesterol 41mg
Sodium 169mg
Total Carbohydrates 2g
Dietary Fiber 3g
Sugars 6g
Protein 20g
Potassium 644mg

55. Chicken Tikka Masala

Serves: 6
Preparation time: 30 minutes
Ingredients:

2 tablespoons butter

1 onion, chopped

½ bell pepper, chopped

3 cloves garlic, minced

1 teaspoon fresh ginger, grated

1 teaspoon turmeric

1 teaspoon cumin

2 teaspoons garam masala

1 teaspoon coriander

¼ teaspoon cayenne pepper

Salt to taste

15 oz. canned diced tomatoes

½ cup coconut milk

2 lb. chicken breast

Preparation:

1) Select the sauté mode in the Instant Pot.
2) Add the butter.
3) Once melted, add the onion and bell pepper.
4) Cook for 4 minutes.
5) Add the garlic, ginger, turmeric, cumin, garam masala, coriander, cayenne pepper and salt. Cook for 1-2 minutes.
6) Pour in the tomatoes and coconut milk. Mix well.
7) Place the chicken on top. Cover the pot and set it to poultry.
8) Release the pressure naturally.
9) Take the chicken out of the pot and shred with forks.
10) Transfer the sauce to a blender. Blend until smooth.
11) Pour the sauce over the chicken before serving.

Serving Suggestion: Serve with fresh green salad.

Tip: An alternative would be to cook the chicken in manual setting. Cook at high pressure for 15 minutes.

Nutritional Information Per Serving:

Calories 280

Total Fat 23g

Saturated Fat 7g

Cholesterol 109mg

Sodium 862mg

Total Carbohydrates 6g

Dietary Fiber 1g

Sugars 2g

Protein 33g

Potassium 792mg

56. ROSEMARY CHICKEN

Serves: 4
Preparation time: 20 minutes
Ingredients:
2 chicken breasts
Salt and pepper to taste
1 cup chicken broth
2 teaspoons fresh rosemary, minced
¼ cup mayo
1 tablespoon green onions, sliced
2 tablespoons almonds, slivered
2 teaspoons lemon juice
Preparation:
1) Season the chicken with the salt and pepper.
2) Add the chicken to the Instant Pot.
3) Pour in the chicken broth.
4) Seal the pot.
5) Set it to manual.
6) Cook at high pressure for 15 minutes.
7) Release the pressure naturally.
8) Take the chicken out of the pot.
9) Shred using a fork.
10) Mix the shredded chicken with the rest of the ingredients.

Serving Suggestion: Serve on top of Romaine lettuce leaves.
Tip: You can also slice the chicken breasts in cubes.
Nutritional Information Per Serving:
Calories 249
Total Fat 15g
Saturated Fat 6g
Cholesterol 65mg
Sodium 199mg
Total Carbohydrates 1g
Protein 22g
Potassium 216mg

57. CHICKEN SHAWARMA

Categories:
Serves: 4
Preparation time: 60 minutes
Ingredients:

1 lb. chicken thigh, sliced
3 teaspoons olive oil, divided
1 teaspoon ground cumin
2 teaspoons dried oregano
1 teaspoon ground coriander
1 teaspoon ground cinnamon

½ teaspoon cayenne
½ teaspoon ground allspice
1 teaspoon salt
1 cup white onion, sliced
1 cup tzatziki sauce

Preparation:

1) Marinate the chicken in a mixture of 1 teaspoon olive oil, cumin, oregano, coriander, cinnamon, cayenne, allspice and salt for 30 minutes.
2) Press the sauté function in the Instant Pot.
3) Add the remaining olive oil.
4) Cook the chicken for 4 minutes, stirring frequently.
5) Pour in ½ cup of water.
6) Scrape the brown bits using a wooden spoon.
7) Add the onion. Seal the pot. Choose manual setting.
8) Cook at high pressure for 10 minutes.
9) Release the pressure quickly.
10) Serve with the tzatziki sauce.

Serving Suggestion: Wrap the chicken shawarma in low carb pita bread or large lettuce leaves.

Tip: If you want to marinate the chicken longer, place in a re-sealable bag and chill in the refrigerator.

Nutritional Information Per Serving:

Calories   264
Total Fat 12.2g
Saturated Fat 2.9g
Cholesterol 101mg
Sodium 681mg

Total Carbohydrate 4.2g
Dietary Fiber 1.4g
Total Sugars 1.3g
Protein 33.4g
Potassium 350mg

58. CHICKEN CARNITAS

Serves: 4
Preparation time: 30 minutes
Ingredients:

2 teaspoons ground cumin
1 teaspoon dried oregano
½ teaspoon ground cinnamon
1 teaspoon chili powder
2 lb. chicken thighs
Salt and pepper to taste

¼ cup orange juice
¼ cup lime juice
4 cloves garlic, minced
1 bay leaf
6 tablespoons olive oil

Preparation:

1) Combine the oregano, cumin, cinnamon and chili powder in a bowl.
2) Season the chicken with the salt and pepper.
3) Sprinkle generously both sides of the chicken with the spice mixture.
4) Pour the orange juice and lime juice into the Instant Pot.
5) Add the chicken. Sprinkle the garlic on top. Add the bay leaf. Seal the pot.
6) Choose manual mode. Cook at high pressure for 8 minutes.
7) Release the pressure quickly.
8) Slice the chicken in cubes.
9) Press the sauté setting in the Instant Pot.
10) Pour in the olive oil.
11) Brown the chicken and serve.

Serving Suggestion: Serve with any of these options: guacamole, sour cream, fresh cilantro, shredded cabbage.

Tip: Use freshly squeezed juices for this recipe.

Nutritional Information Per Serving:

Calories   630
Total Fat 38.2g
Saturated Fat 7.7g
Cholesterol 202mg
Sodium 204mg
Total Carbohydrate 3.9g
Dietary Fiber 0.7g
Total Sugars 1.4g
Protein 66.2g
Potassium 633mg

59. Buffalo Chicken with Cauliflower

Serves: 6
Preparation time: 30 minutes
Ingredients:
2 cups chicken, cooked and sliced into cubes
1 head cauliflower, chopped
¼ cup ranch dressing
½ cup buffalo sauce
Salt and pepper to taste
½ cup cream cheese, cubed
2 cups cheddar cheese, shredded
Preparation:
1) Add the chicken, cauliflower, ranch dressing, buffalo sauce, salt and pepper in the Instant Pot.
2) Mix well.
3) Cover the pot.
4) Choose manual mode.
5) Cook at high pressure for 5 minutes.
6) Release the pressure quickly.
7) Stir in the cream cheese and top with the cheddar before serving.

Serving Suggestion: Garnish with chopped parsley or dried basil.

Tip: You can also cook the chicken in the Instant Pot by using the sauté function.

Nutritional Information Per Serving:
Calories 344
Total fat 24.8g
Saturated Fat 12.4g
Cholesterol 100mg
Sodium 778.8mg
Carbohydrates 7.7g
Fiber 2.3g
Total Sugars 3g
Protein 23.8g
Potassium 290.3mg

60. CHICKEN ADOBO SHREDS

Serves: 4
Preparation time: 30 minutes
Ingredients:

4 chicken breasts

Garlic salt and pepper to taste

3 tablespoons olive oil

1 onion, chopped

3 cloves garlic, crushed

¼ cup soy sauce

1 cup chicken stock

3 tablespoons vinegar

2 bay leaves

Preparation:

1) Season the chicken breasts with the garlic salt and pepper.
2) Pour the olive oil into the Instant Pot.
3) Press sauté.
4) Add the chicken and cook until brown on both sides.
5) Add the onion, garlic, soy sauce, chicken stock, vinegar and bay leaves.
6) Cover the pot.
7) Set it to manual.
8) Cook at high pressure for 15 minutes.
9) Release the pressure naturally.
10) Take the chicken out.
11) Shred using a fork.

Serving Suggestion: Enjoy this dish with a cup of cauliflower rice.

Tip: You can also sauté the onion and garlic first before pressure cooking.

Nutritional Information Per Serving:

Calories   420

Total Fat 21.5g

Saturated Fat 4.5g

Cholesterol 130mg

Sodium 392mg

Total Carbohydrate 8.4g

Dietary Fiber 1.2g

Total Sugars 2.5g

Protein 46.9g

Potassium 554mg

Chapter 14: 20 Keto Diet Fish & Seafood Recipes

61. Garlic Mussels

Serves: 4-6
Preparation time: 20 minutes
Ingredients:

4 tablespoons butter
1 shallot, minced
5 cloves garlic, crushed and minced

2 lb. mussels, scrubbed and debearded
1 tablespoon lemon juice
1 cup chicken stock

Preparation:

1) Select the sauté setting in the Instant Pot.
2) Add the butter.
3) Once melted, add the shallot and garlic.
4) Cook for 1-2 minutes.
5) Add the mussels to the pot.
6) Pour in the lemon juice and chicken stock.
7) Cover the pot.
8) Set it to manual mode.
9) Cook at high pressure for 3 minutes.
10) Release the pressure quickly.
11) Pour the sauce over the mussels before serving.

Serving Suggestion: Sprinkle with chopped fresh parsley before serving.

Tip: Use freshly squeezed lemon juice. Discard any mussels that are open prior to cooking, and those that did not open after cooking.

Nutritional Information Per Serving:

Calories   306
Total Fat 16.8g
Saturated Fat 8.3g
Cholesterol 94mg
Sodium 923mg
Total Carbohydrate 9.9g
Dietary Fiber 0.1g
Total Sugars 0.3g
Protein 27.6g
Potassium 753mg

62. Salmon in Lemon Sauce

Serves: 3
Preparation time: 15 minutes
Ingredients:
8 oz. salmon fillet
2 teaspoons lemon juice
1 teaspoon lemon zest
2 tablespoons alternative sweetener
Salt and pepper to taste
1 tablespoon butter
Preparation:
1) Season the salmon fillet with lemon juice, lemon zest, sweetener, salt, pepper and butter.
2) Wrap the salmon in foil.
3) Add ½ cup water to the Instant Pot.
4) Place the wrapped salmon inside the pot.
5) Close the pot.
6) Choose the manual mode.
7) Cook it at high pressure for 5 minutes.
8) Release the pressure naturally.
9) Unwrap the foil.
10) Pour the juices over the salmon before serving.

Serving Suggestion: Sprinkle chopped parsley on top of the salmon.

Tip: You can also do this recipe using other types of fish like cod or tuna.

Nutritional Information Per Serving:
Calories   235
Total Fat 12.5g
Saturated Fat 5.1g
Cholesterol 44mg
Sodium 61mg
Total Carbohydrate 0.2g
Dietary Fiber 0.1g
Total Sugars 0.1g
Protein 14.8g
Potassium 298mg

63. Salmon in Chili Lime Sauce

Serves: 2
Preparation time: 15 minutes
Ingredients:

2 salmon fillets

Salt and pepper to taste

1 tablespoon honey

1 jalapeno, seeded and diced

1 tablespoon lime juice

2 cloves garlic, crushed and minced

1 tablespoon olive oil

½ teaspoon cumin

½ teaspoon paprika

1 tablespoon fresh parsley

Preparation:

1) Rub the salmon fillets with the salt and pepper.
2) Pour 1 cup of water into the Instant Pot.
3) Add a steamer basket to the pot.
4) Place the salmon on top of the basket.
5) Cover the pot.
6) Choose the steam mode.
7) Release the pressure quickly.
8) Mix the rest of the ingredients in a bowl.
9) Pour over the salmon before serving.

Serving Suggestion: Top with chopped chives.

Tip: Use vegetable broth in place of water.

Nutritional Information Per Serving:

Calories 400

Total Fat 25g

Saturated Fat 5g

Cholesterol 78mg

Sodium 90mg

Total Carbohydrates 10.5g

Dietary Fiber 0.5g

Sugars 9g

Protein 29g

Potassium 580mg

64. SALMON & ASPARAGUS

Serves: 4
Preparation time: 20 minutes
Ingredients:

2 cloves garlic, crushed

4 sprigs fresh dill

1 lb. salmon fillet

1 tablespoon avocado oil

3 teaspoons butter, divided

Salt to taste

1 teaspoon garlic powder

½ teaspoon dried thyme

6 lemon slices

1 bundle asparagus, sliced

Preparation:

1) Add 1 cup of water to the Instant Pot.
2) Add the garlic and fresh dill.
3) Place a steamer basket inside the pot.
4) Put the salmon on top of the basket.
5) Spread the avocado oil and 1 teaspoon butter on the salmon fillet.
6) Sprinkle both sides with the salt, garlic powder and thyme.
7) Top with the lemon slices.
8) Close the pot.
9) Set it to manual.
10) Cook at high pressure for 4 minutes.
11) Release the pressure quickly.
12) Transfer the salmon on a plate.
13) Cover with foil.
14) Press the sauté setting in the Instant Pot.
15) Add the asparagus.
16) Cook for 4-5 minutes.
17) Season with the salt.

Serving Suggestion: Sprinkle grated parmesan on top.

Tip: If dill is not available, you can use basil, thyme or tarragon.

Nutritional Information Per Serving:

Calories   193

Total Fat 10.4g

Saturated Fat 2.9g

Cholesterol 58mg

Sodium 113mg

Total Carbohydrate 3.2g

Dietary Fiber 1.1g

Total Sugars 0.8g

Protein 23g

Potassium 529mg

65. LEMON PEPPER FISH

Serves: 4
Preparation time: 15 minutes
Ingredients:

5 sprigs fresh tarragon
1 lb. white fish fillet
3 teaspoons ghee, divided
Salt and pepper to taste

4 lemon slices
1 tablespoon butter
1 zucchini, sliced into strips
1 red bell pepper, sliced into strips

Preparation:

1) Add ¾ cup of water in the Instant Pot.
2) Add the fresh tarragon.
3) Place a steamer rack inside.
4) Put the fish on top.
5) Coat the fish with ghee.
6) Season with the salt and pepper.
7) Top with the lemon slices.
8) Seal the pot.
9) Choose the steam setting.
10) Release the pressure quickly.
11) Remove the fish from the pot.
12) Discard the water.
13) Press the sauté setting.
14) Add the butter.
15) Cook the vegetables for 2 minutes.
16) Serve the fish with the vegetables.

Serving Suggestion: Serve with a cup of fresh cilantro
Tip: Tarragon may be replaced with parsley or dill.
Nutritional Information Per Serving:

Calories   268
Total Fat 14.8g
Saturated Fat 5.1g
Cholesterol 103mg
Sodium 100mg

Total Carbohydrate 4.6g
Dietary Fiber 1.2g
Total Sugars 2.5g
Protein 28.8g
Potassium 656mg

66. SEAFOOD GUMBO

Serves: 8
Preparation time: 10 minutes
Ingredients:

3 tablespoons avocado oil
24 oz. sea bass fillet, sliced into bite-sized pieces
3 tablespoons creole seasoning
2 onions, diced
4 ribs celery, diced
2 bell peppers, diced

1 ½ cups bone broth
28 oz. diced tomatoes
¼ cup tomato paste
3 bay leaves
2 lb. shrimp, peeled and deveined
Salt and pepper to taste

Preparation:

1) Set the Instant Pot to sauté.
2) Pour in the avocado oil.
3) Cook the sea bass for 3 minutes per side.
4) Transfer the fish to a platter.
5) Add the onion, celery and bell pepper.
6) Put the fish back to the pot.
7) Add the broth, tomatoes, tomato paste, and bay leaves.
8) Stir in the shrimp.
9) Season with the salt and pepper.
10) Seal the pot.
11) Set it to manual.
12) Cook at high pressure for 10 minutes.
13) Release the pressure quickly.
14) Discard the bay leaves before serving.

Serving Suggestion: Garnish with chopped parsley.

Tip: You can also use other types of fish such as tuna or salmon.

Nutritional Information Per Serving:

Calories 292
Total Fat 15.1g
Saturated Fat 8.3g
Cholesterol 284mg
Sodium 1581mg

Total Carbohydrate 7.3g
Dietary Fiber 2.8g
Total Sugars 4.3g
Protein 47.8g
Potassium 902mg

67. CREAMY SPICY SHRIMP

Serves: 6
Preparation time: 15 minutes
Ingredients:

2 tablespoons butter
4 cloves garlic, minced
½ teaspoons red pepper flakes
1 lb. shrimp, frozen
Salt and pepper to taste

½ teaspoons paprika
2 cups low carb pasta (uncooked)
1 cup chicken broth
½ cup half and half

Preparation:

1) Add the butter to the Instant Pot.
2) Press the sauté function.
3) Wait for the butter to melt.
4) Add the garlic and pepper flakes.
5) Cook for 2 minutes.
6) Add the shrimp.
7) Season with the salt, pepper and paprika.
8) Add the pasta and broth.
9) Cover the pot.
10) Set it to manual.
11) Cook at high pressure for 2 minutes.
12) Release the pressure quickly.
13) Press the sauté button.
14) Stir in the half and half.

Serving Suggestion: Sprinkle with parmesan on top.

Tip: You can omit the pasta and serve with spaghetti squash instead.

Nutritional Information Per Serving:

Calories   312
Total Fat 18g
Saturated Fat 7g
Cholesterol 213mg
Sodium 921mg

Total Carbohydrate 9g
Dietary Fiber 2g
Total Sugars 1g
Protein 24g
Potassium 197mg

68. SHRIMP IN COCONUT MILK

Serves: 4
Preparation time: 20 minutes
Ingredients:

1 lb. shrimp, peeled and deveined
1 tablespoon ginger, minced
1 tablespoon garlic, minced
½ teaspoon turmeric

1 teaspoon salt
½ teaspoon cayenne pepper
1 teaspoon garam masala
½ cup coconut milk

Preparation:

1) Combine all the ingredients.
2) Pour into a baking dish.
3) Pour 2 cups of water into the Instant Pot.
4) Place a steamer rack inside the pot.
5) Put the baking dish on top of the rack.
6) Cover the dish with foil.
7) Seal the pot.
8) Set it to manual.
9) Cook at low pressure for 4 minutes.

Serving Suggestion: Sprinkle with chopped fresh chives.

Tip: Use unsweetened coconut milk if possible.

Nutritional Information Per Serving:

Calories   192
Total Fat 12g
Saturated Fat 9g
Cholesterol 209mg
Sodium 921mg
Total Carbohydrate 4g
Dietary Fiber 2g
Total Sugars 1.2g
Protein 19g
Potassium 216mg

69. MUSSELS WITH SPICY MAYO

Serves: 4-6
Preparation time: 50 minutes
Ingredients:
2 cloves garlic, crushed and minced
3 tomatoes, chopped
1 cup white wine
1 bay leaf
2 lb. mussels, scrubbed and debearded
½ cup parsley, chopped
¼ cup mayonnaise
2 tablespoons roasted red pepper, minced
Preparation:
1) Add the garlic, tomatoes, wine and bay leave in the Instant Pot.
2) Place the mussels on top.
3) Seal the pot.
4) Choose the manual mode.
5) Cook at high pressure for 3 minutes.
6) Release the pressure quickly.
7) In a bowl, mix the parsley, mayo and red pepper.
8) Serve the mussels with the spicy mayo dip.
Serving Suggestion: Garnish with lemon or lime wedges.
Tip: Try adding steamed spinach to the dish.
Nutritional Information Per Serving:
Calories   216
Total Fat 6.8g
Saturated Fat 1.2g
Cholesterol 45mg
Sodium 520mg
Total Carbohydrate 12.3g
Dietary Fiber 1g
Total Sugars 2.8g
Protein 18.9g
Potassium 708mg

70. Shrimp Paella

Serves: 4
Preparation time: 15 minutes
Ingredients:

1 lb. shrimp, peeled
4 tablespoons butter
4 cups cauliflower rice
1 onion, chopped
4 cloves garlic, chopped
½ cup white wine
1 cup chicken broth

1 pinch saffron threads
1 teaspoon paprika
1 red pepper, chopped
Salt and pepper to taste
1 teaspoon turmeric
¼ teaspoon red pepper flakes

Preparation:

1) Choose the sauté setting in the Instant Pot.
2) Add the butter.
3) Cook the onion and garlic for 2-3 minutes.
4) Add the rest of the ingredients except the cauliflower rice.
5) Cover the pot.
6) Set it to manual.
7) Cook at high pressure for 5 minutes.
8) Release the pressure quickly.
9) Stir in the cauliflower rice before serving.

Serving Suggestion: Serve with cilantro or green salad.
Nutritional Information Per Serving:

Calories 318
Total Fat 23.2g
Saturated Fat 5g
Cholesterol 253.3 mg
Sodium 790 mg
Total Carbohydrate 4.7g
Dietary Fiber 2.1 g
Sugars 0.5 g
Protein 26.4 g

71. Salmon in Creamy Herb Sauce

Serves: 4
Preparation time: 20 minutes
Ingredients:

1 teaspoon garlic, minced
4 salmon fillets
½ cup heavy cream
1 teaspoon lemon juice
1 cup parmesan cheese, grated

1 tablespoon fresh dill
1 tablespoon fresh chives, chopped
1 tablespoon fresh parsley, chopped
Salt and pepper to taste

Preparation:

1) Pour ½ cup of water into the Instant Pot.
2) Add the garlic.
3) Place the steamer rack inside the pot.
4) Put the salmon on the rack.
5) Cover the pot.
6) Set it to manual.
7) Cook at high pressure for 5 minutes.
8) Release the pressure quickly.
9) Transfer the salmon to a plate.
10) Remove the steamer rack.
11) Press the sauté setting.
12) Stir in the heavy cream.
13) Simmer for 3 minutes.
14) Add the rest of the ingredients before serving.

Serving Suggestion: Serve with buttered vegetables.

Tip: Make sure that you use freshly squeezed lemon juice.

Nutritional Information Per Serving:

Calories   314
Total Fat 18.1g
Saturated Fat 6g
Cholesterol 104mg
Sodium 152mg

Total Carbohydrate 1.5g
Dietary Fiber 0.2g
Total Sugars 0.1g
Protein 37.4g
Potassium 733mg

72. Lobster Fondue

Serves: 2
Preparation time: 30 minutes
Ingredients:

2 lobster tails

1 tablespoon butter

2 oz. smoked bacon

1 clove garlic, sliced

1 cup breadcrumbs

¼ cup parmesan, grated

8 oz. low carb pasta

1 cup dry white wine

Salt and pepper to taste

1 clove garlic, grated

¾ cup evaporated milk

1 tablespoon cherry brandy

Preparation:

1) Pour 1 cup of water into the Instant Pot. Place a steamer basket inside.
2) Add the lobster tails. Cover the pot. Set it to manual.
3) Cook at low pressure for 3 minutes. Do a quick pressure release.
4) Soak the lobster tails in a bowl of ice water. Remove the shell.
5) Chop the lobster meat.   Place in a bowl and set aside.
6) Remove the water and steamer basket from the pot.
7) Add the bacon and cook until crispy.
8) Remove the bacon and set aside.
9) Add the sliced garlic and cook for 30 seconds. Add the butter. Stir in the breadcrumbs.
10) Fold in the parmesan. Remove from heat and set aside.
11) Add the pasta, wine, salt, pepper ½ cup of water and grated garlic in the Instant Pot.
12) Cover the pot and cook at high pressure for 5 minutes.
13) Release the pressure quickly.
14) Choose the sauté function.
15) Pour in the evaporated milk and cherry brandy.
16) Add the lobster meat and stir until creamy.
17) Serve in bowls. Top with the bacon mixture.

Serving Suggestion: Garnish with fresh chives.

Tip: To save time, you can use prepared lobster meat.

Nutritional Information Per Serving:

Calories   756

Total Fat 38.2g

Saturated Fat 12.7g

Cholesterol 282mg

Sodium 982mg

Total Carbohydrate 8.3g

Dietary Fiber 2.5g

Total Sugars 9g

Protein 53.2g

Potassium 869mg

73. SALMON & SPINACH PESTO

Serves: 4
Preparation time: 30 minutes
Ingredients:

2 cloves garlic

¼ cup walnuts

10 cups baby spinach

1 cup parmesan, grated

½ cup olive oil

Salt and pepper to taste

1 tablespoon butter

16 oz. low carb pasta

12 oz. smoked salmon, sliced

1 ½ cup heavy cream, divided

1 teaspoon lemon zest, grated

1 teaspoon lemon juice

Preparation:

1) Add the garlic, walnuts, spinach, parmesan, olive oil, salt and pepper in a food processor.
2) Pulse until pureed.
3) Choose the manual setting in the Instant Pot.
4) Pour in 4 cups of water.
5) Add the butter and pasta.
6) Cover the pot.
7) Choose manual setting.
8) Cook at high pressure for 4 minutes.
9) Release the pressure quickly.
10) Select the sauté setting.
11) Add the rest of the ingredients.
12) Mix well.
13) Simmer for 1-2 minutes.

Serving Suggestion: Sprinkle with more parmesan cheese on top before serving.
Tip: Use basil in place of spinach if you prefer the traditional pesto flavor.
Nutritional Information Per Serving:

Calories   667

Total Fat 58.8g

Saturated Fat 18.4g

Cholesterol 94mg

Sodium 934mg

Total Carbohydrate 8.7g

Dietary Fiber 3.3g

Total Sugars 2.5g

Protein 24.9g

Potassium 652mg

74. Asian Tuna

Serves: 2
Preparation time: 15 minutes
Ingredients:

1 tablespoon coconut oil

1 tablespoon brown sugar

2 tablespoon maple syrup

1 teaspoon paprika

3 tablespoon coconut aminos

¼ teaspoon ginger, grated

2 tuna fillets

Salt and pepper to taste

Preparation:

1) Select the sauté setting in the Instant Pot.
2) Add the coconut oil and brown sugar.
3) Cook until the sugar has been dissolved.
4) Pour in the maple syrup, paprika, coconut aminos and ginger.
5) Mix well.
6) Place the tuna fillets on top.
7) Season with the salt and pepper.
8) Cover the pot.
9) Set it to manual.
10) Cook at low pressure for 2 minutes.
11) Release the pressure naturally.

Serving Suggestion: Sprinkle sesame seeds and chopped fresh scallions on top before serving.

Tip: You can also use other types of fish for this recipe.

Nutritional Information Per Serving:

Calories   150

Total Fat 17.8g

Saturated Fat 6.1g

Cholesterol 3mg

Sodium 8mg

Total Carbohydrate 8.5g

Dietary Fiber 0.4g

Total Sugars 16.4g

Protein 2.8g

Potassium 105mg

75. Fish Croquettes

Serves: 2
Preparation time: 20 minutes
Ingredients:

2 salmon fillets

Salt and pepper to taste

1 egg, beaten

¼ cup onion, chopped

2 stalks green onion, sliced

1 cup panko breadcrumbs

2 tablespoons olive oil

Preparation:

1) Pour 1 cup of water into the Instant Pot.
2) Place a steamer rack inside.
3) Add the salmon fillets on top.
4) Season both sides with the salt and pepper.
5) Cover the pot.
6) Set it to manual.
7) Cook at high pressure for 3 minutes.
8) Release the pressure quickly.
9) Take the fish out.
10) Shred the fish and add the egg, onion and green onion.
11) Add the breadcrumbs.
12) Form into patties.
13) Remove the rack and water from the pot.
14) Pour in the olive oil.
15) Add the fish patties.
16) Cook until golden.

Serving Suggestion: Serve with tartar sauce.

Tip: You can also use tuna or halibut.

Nutritional Information Per Serving:

Calories   433

Total Fat 27.5g

Saturated Fat 4.3g

Cholesterol 160mg

Sodium 181mg

Total Carbohydrate 10.1g

Dietary Fiber 1.7g

Total Sugars 1.4g

Protein 38.7g

Potassium 776mg

76. Shrimp & Vegetable Risotto

Serves: 4
Preparation time: 30 minutes
Ingredients:

2 teaspoons olive oil

1 bunch asparagus, sliced

3 garlic cloves, minced

½ onion, chopped

1 tablespoon butter

½ cup dry white wine

3 ½ cups chicken broth

½ cup parmesan cheese, shredded

Salt and pepper to taste

1 lb. shrimp, peeled and deveined

1 cup fresh spinach

1 tablespoon parsley, chopped

4 cups cauliflower rice

1 tablespoon lemon juice

Preparation:

1) Set the Instant Pot to sauté. Pour in half of the olive oil.
2) Cook the asparagus for 3 minutes.
3) Add the garlic and onion. Cook for 1 minute.
4) Add the butter and stir well.
5) Deglaze the pot by pouring in the white wine.
6) Add the chicken broth and parmesan. Stir well.
7) Season with the salt and pepper.   Cover the pot.
8) Set tit to manual.
9) Cook at high pressure for 8 minutes.
10) While waiting, season the shrimp with salt and pepper.
11) Release the pressure quickly.
12) Stir in the shrimp and vegetables.
13) Press sauté function. Cook for 4 minutes.
14) Stir in the cauliflower rice and drizzle with the lemon juice before serving.

Serving Suggestion: Garnish with chopped parsley.

Tip: You can also add other seafood such as squid or fish flakes.

Nutritional Information Per Serving:

Calories   277

Total Fat 9.9g

Saturated Fat 4.1g

Cholesterol 251mg

Sodium 1040mg

Total Carbohydrate 6.8g

Dietary Fiber 1g

Total Sugars 1.9g

Protein 33.4g

Potassium 524mg

77. SALMON & VEGGIES WITH SPICY MAYO

Serves: 2
Preparation time: 20 minutes
Ingredients:

2 salmon fillets
¼ teaspoon chili powder
¼ teaspoon smoked paprika
¼ teaspoon onion powder
Salt and pepper to taste
1 cup broccoli florets

1 cup cauliflower florets
1 bell pepper, sliced
1 onion, sliced
1 tablespoon mayonnaise
1 tablespoon hot sauce

Preparation:

1) Pour 1 cup of water into the Instant Pot.
2) Add a steamer rack inside.
3) Place salmon fillets on top.
4) Season the fish with chili powder, paprika, onion powder, salt and pepper.
5) Top with the vegetables.
6) Sprinkle salt and pepper on the veggies.
7) Close the pot.
8) Set it to manual.
9) Cook at high pressure for 6 minutes.
10) Do a quick pressure release.
11) Mix mayo and hot sauce.
12) Serve salmon and veggies with the spicy mayo sauce.

Serving Suggestion: Sprinkle chopped fresh oregano.

Tip: You can also use homemade chili paste in place of the hot sauce.

Nutritional Information Per Serving:

Calories   337
Total Fat 14g
Saturated Fat 2g
Cholesterol 80mg
Sodium 358mg
Total Carbohydrate 17.8g
Dietary Fiber 4.7g
Total Sugars 8g
Protein 38.2g
Potassium 1198mg

78. Shrimp Alfredo

Serves: 4
Preparation time: 20 minutes
Ingredients:
1 tablespoon olive oil
¼ cup onion, diced
4 cups frozen shrimp
2 cups chicken stock
2 cups low carb pasta
1 cup parmesan cheese, grated
1 cup half and half
Salt and pepper to taste
Preparation:
1) Press the sauté function in the Instant Pot.
2) Pour in the olive oil.
3) Add the onion.
4) Cook for 5 minutes.
5) Add the shrimp, stock, and pasta.
6) Seal the pot.
7) Set it to manual.
8) Cook at high pressure for 7 minutes.
9) Release the pressure quickly.
10) Press the sauté button.
11) Stir in the rest of the ingredients.

Serving Suggestion: Sprinkle with chopped chives.
Nutritional Information Per Serving:
Calories   369
Total Fat 12.8g
Saturated Fat 5.9g
Cholesterol 70mg
Sodium 514mg
Total Carbohydrate 4.2g
Dietary Fiber 0.2g
Total Sugars 0.8g
Protein 10.2g
Potassium 97mg

79. SHRIMP MAC & CHEESE

Serves: 2
Preparation time: 20 minutes
Ingredients:

1 tablespoon butter

¼ red pepper, sliced

¼ green pepper, sliced

1 ¼ cups low carb macaroni pasta

15 shrimps, peeled and deveined

1 tablespoon Cajun spice

½ cup cheddar cheese, shredded

2/3 cup coconut milk

Preparation:

1) Choose the sauté function in the Instant Pot.
2) Add the butter.
3) Cook the peppers for 1 minute.
4) Add the pasta.
5) Pour in 2 cups of water.
6) Cover the pot.
7) Set it to manual.
8) Cook at high pressure for 3 minutes.
9) Do a quick pressure release.
10) Press the sauté mode.
11) Add the shrimp.
12) Cook for 2 minutes.
13) Stir in the rest of the ingredients before serving.

Serving Suggestion: Garnish with peeled shrimp and chopped parsley.

Tip: Use keto-friendly low carb macaroni pasta for this recipe.

Nutritional Information Per Serving:

Calories   459

Total Fat 22.2g

Saturated Fat 11.8g

Cholesterol 399mg

Sodium 902mg

Total Carbohydrate 7.1g

Dietary Fiber 1.1g

Total Sugars 6.2g

Protein 48.9g

Potassium 410mg

80. Steamed Clams in Garlic Butter Sauce

Serves: 4
Preparation time: 25 minutes
Ingredients:

1 stick butter, divided
¼ lb. radish, scrubbed, trimmed and sliced
12 cloves garlic, minced
1 cup dry white wine

Salt to taste
5 lb. clams, scrubbed and trimmed
1 tablespoon lemon juice
½ cup parsley, chopped

Preparation:

1) Press sauté in the Instant Pot.
2) Add half of the butter and radish.
3) Cook for 2 minutes.
4) Add the garlic and cook for 1 minute.
5) Pour in the white wine.
6) Reduce for 3 minutes.
7) Season with the salt.
8) Add the clams.
9) Cover the pot.
10) Choose the steam setting.
11) Set it to 1 minute.
12) Release the pressure naturally.
13) Remove the radish and clams.
14) Transfer to a bowl.
15) Select the sauté mode.
16) Simmer the sauce for 5 minutes.
17) Add the remaining butter, parsley and lemon juice.
18) Pour the sauce over the clams and radish before serving.

Serving Suggestion: Serve with green leafy salad or cauliflower rice.

Tip: Discard clams that are already open prior to cooking or those that did not open after cooking.

Nutritional Information Per Serving:

Calories 559
Total Fat 24.3g
Saturated Fat 14.6g
Cholesterol 61mg
Sodium 2308mg

Total Carbohydrate 7.1g
Dietary Fiber 4.5g
Total Sugars 6.6g
Protein 5.3g
Potassium 916mg

Chapter 15: 10 Keto Diet Vegan & Vegetarian Recipes

81. Cabbage in Cream Sauce

Serves: 4-6
Preparation time: 20 minutes
Ingredients:

1 tablespoon olive oil
1 onion, chopped
1 cup bacon, diced
2 cups bone broth
4 cups cabbage, chopped
1 bay leaf
¼ teaspoon nutmeg
1 cup coconut milk
Salt to taste

Preparation:

1) Choose the sauté function in the Instant Pot. Pour in the olive oil.
2) Add the onion and cook until soft. Add the bacon and cook until golden crisp.
3) Pour in the bone broth. Scrape the bottom of the pot using a wooden spoon.
4) Add the cabbage and bay leaf. Cover the pot.
5) Press the manual mode. Cook at high pressure for 4 minutes.
6) Release the pressure naturally.
7) Press the sauté function.
8) Stir in the coconut milk.
9) Season with the salt and nutmeg.
10) Simmer for 5 minutes.

Serving Suggestion: Sprinkle parsley flakes on top.

Tip: You can also add other vegetables like young corn or spinach if you like.

Nutritional Information Per Serving:

Calories   699
Total Fat 84.3g
Saturated Fat 35.1g
Cholesterol 175mg
Sodium 380mg
Total Carbohydrate 12.4g
Dietary Fiber 3.8g
Total Sugars 5.5g
Protein 71.4g
Potassium 1360mg

82. Spinach & Mushroom Curry

Serves: 4
Preparation time: 20 minutes
Ingredients:

2 tablespoons olive oil
3 cloves garlic, minced
1 teaspoon cumin seeds
1 onion, chopped
1 jalapeño, sliced into quarter
3 tomatoes, chopped
1 tablespoon coriander powder

1 teaspoon garam masala
¼ teaspoon red chili powder
1 teaspoon turmeric powder
9 oz. spinach, chopped
8 oz. mushrooms, sliced
Salt to taste

Preparation:

1) Select the sauté mode in the Instant Pot.
2) Pour in the olive oil.
3) Add the garlic and cumin seeds.
4) Cook for 1 minute.
5) Add the onion and jalapeno.
6) Cook for 3 minutes.
7) Add the tomatoes and spice powders.
8) Add the rest of the ingredients.
9) Mix well.
10) Cover the pot.
11) Set it to manual.
12) Cook at high pressure for 3 minutes.
13) Release the pressure quickly.
14) Set it to sauté function.
15) Simmer until sauce is reduced.

Serving Suggestion: Serve with a cup of cauliflower rice.

Tip: Use curry powder if garam masala or coriander powder is not available.

Nutritional Information Per Serving:

Calories   245
Total Fat 25.7g
Saturated Fat 5.2g
Cholesterol 0mg
Sodium 205mg

Total Carbohydrate 9.5g
Dietary Fiber 3.9g
Total Sugars 5.8g
Protein 10.1g
Potassium 1664mg

83. Radishes with Soy Sauce & Sesame Seeds

Serves: 4
Preparation time: 15 minutes
Ingredients:

2 tablespoons olive oil

4 cups radishes, sliced

1 ½ tablespoons soy sauce

1 teaspoon sesame oil

2 teaspoons black sesame seeds

Preparation:

1) Press the sauté function in the Instant Pot.
2) Add the oil.
3) Add the radishes and cook until a little brown.
4) Add the rest of the ingredients except the black sesame seeds.
5) Mix well.
6) Cover the pot.
7) Set it to manual.
8) Cook at high pressure for 5 minutes.
9) Release the pressure quickly.
10) Sprinkle with the sesame seeds before serving.

Serving Suggestion: Garnish with chopped chives.

Tip: Sesame oil is optional but is added for a more enticing flavour.

Nutritional Information Per Serving:

Calories   200

Total Fat 17.5g

Saturated Fat 2.9g

Cholesterol 0mg

Sodium 767mg

Total Carbohydrate 9.5g

Dietary Fiber 4.2g

Total Sugars 4.5g

Protein 2.9g

Potassium 581mg

84. Spaghetti Squash in Alfredo Sauce

Serves: 6
Preparation time: 15 minutes
Ingredients:

1 whole spaghetti squash, sliced crosswise and seeded

3 teaspoons olive oil

16 oz. chicken breast, sliced into cubes

Salt and pepper to taste

1 tablespoon garlic, minced

½ cup chicken broth

¼ cup heavy whipping cream

2 cups almond milk

¾ tablespoon butter, softened

4 oz. cream cheese, softened

1 cup parmesan cheese, shredded

2 cups broccoli, chopped

1 tablespoon almond flour

Preparation:

1) Pour 1 cup of water into the Instant Pot.
2) Place the spaghetti squash inside with the sliced side up. Cover the pot.
3) Set it to manual. Cook at high pressure for 7 minutes.
4) Release the pressure quickly.
5) Take out the squash and shred using a fork. Discard the water.
6) Set the Instant Pot to sauté.
7) Season the chicken cubes with the salt and pepper. Pour in the olive oil.
8) Add the chicken and cook until brown on both sides.
9) Add the garlic and cook for 1 minute.
10) Pour in the chicken broth.
11) Scrape the brown bits from the bottom of the pot using a wooden spoon.
12) Add the cream, milk, butter and cream cheese. Mix well.
13) Add the Parmesan and broccoli.
14) Cook for 2-3 minutes.
15) Stir in the flour to thicken the sauce.
16) Pour the sauce over the pasta before serving.

Serving Suggestion: Garnish with chopped basil or parsley.

Tip: You can skip the flour and simply simmer to thicken the sauce.

Nutritional Information Per Serving:

Calories   462

Total Fat 33.9g

Saturated Fat 23.6g

Cholesterol 80mg

Sodium 230mg

Total Carbohydrate 12g

Dietary Fiber 5.5g

Total Sugars 8.5g

Protein 22.2g

Potassium 879mg

85. LIME CAULIFLOWER RICE

Serves: 4
Preparation time: 20 minutes
Ingredients:
1 head cauliflower, chopped into florets
2 tablespoons coconut oil
1 teaspoon lime juice
Preparation:
1) Pour 1 cup of water into the Instant Pot.
2) Place a steamer rack inside the pot.
3) Put the cauliflower florets on top of the rack.
4) Cover the pot.
5) Press the manual button.
6) Cook at high pressure for 1 minute.
7) Release the pressure quickly.
8) Discard the water and drain the cauliflower.
9) Mash the cauliflower into rice-like consistency.
10) Choose the sauté function in the Instant Pot.
11) Pour in the coconut oil.
12) Add the cauliflower rice to the pot.
13) Cook for 2-3 minutes, stirring frequently.
14) Stir in the lime juice before serving.

Serving Suggestion: Place fresh cilantro sprigs on top of the cauliflower rice.
Tip: Use a potato masher to turn the cauliflower florets into rice.
Nutritional Information Per Serving:
Calories   156
Total Fat 13.7g
Saturated Fat 11.8g
Cholesterol 0mg
Sodium 40mg
Total Carbohydrate 8.9g
Dietary Fiber 3.4g   1
Total Sugars 3.6g
Protein 2.7g
Potassium 427mg

86. Spiced Cauliflower

Serves: 4
Preparation time: 15 minutes
Ingredients:
3 curry leaves
2 teaspoons mustard seeds
4 cups cauliflower florets
1 tablespoon ginger-garlic paste
Salt and pepper to taste
Preparation:
1) Choose sauté mode in your Instant Pot.
2) Coat it with cooking spray.
3) Cook the curry leaves and mustard seeds.
4) Add the cauliflower florets.
5) Season with the salt, pepper and ginger garlic paste.
6) Pour in 1 cup of water.
7) Secure the lid.
8) Choose manual function.
9) Cook at high pressure for 3 minutes.
10) Release the pressure quickly.

Serving Suggestion: Serve as side dish to any meat or seafood main course.

Tip: Use cumin seeds if you do not have mustard seeds.
Nutritional Information Per Serving:
Calories   126
Total Fat 5.9g
Saturated Fat 0.2g
Cholesterol 0mg
Sodium 62mg
Total Carbohydrate 15.7g
Dietary Fiber 6.5g
Total Sugars 5.1g
Protein 5.6g
Potassium 675mg

87. CREAMED SPINACH & MUSTARD LEAVES

Categories:
Serves: 4
Preparation time: 30 minutes
Ingredients:

2 tablespoons ghee

2 onions, diced

2 teaspoons ginger, minced

4 teaspoons garlic, minced

1 teaspoon garam masala

1 teaspoon ground cumin

2 teaspoons salt

1 teaspoon coriander

½ teaspoon turmeric

½ teaspoon cayenne pepper

½ teaspoon black pepper

1 lb. spinach

1 lb. mustard leaves

Preparation:

1) Choose the sauté function in the Instant Pot.
2) Add the ghee.
3) Cook the onion, ginger, garlic and all the spices for 3 minutes, stirring frequently.
4) Add the spinach and mustard greens.
5) Cover the pot.
6) Set it to manual.
7) Cook at high pressure for 15 minutes.
8) Release the pressure naturally.
9) Transfer contents to a blender.
10) Blend until smooth.

Serving Suggestion: Stir in the fenugreek leaves and serve with butter.

Tip: You can choose which spices you'd like to include in the recipe.

Nutritional Information Per Serving:

Calories   167

Total Fat 12.9g

Saturated Fat 7.7g

Cholesterol 32mg

Sodium 1299mg

Total Carbohydrate 11.5g

Dietary Fiber 4.1g

Total Sugars 2.9g

Protein 4.4g

Potassium 764mg

88. Veggie Risotto

Serves: 6-8
Preparation time: 35 minutes
Ingredients:

1 tablespoon olive oil

3 tablespoons butter, cubed and divided

½ onion, chopped

Salt and pepper to taste

½ teaspoon red pepper flakes, crushed

2 cloves garlic, minced

8 oz. asparagus, trimmed and chopped

8 oz. mushrooms, chopped

2 cups baby spinach

½ cup fresh peas

½ cup cheddar cheese, shredded

¼ cup Parmesan cheese, grated

¼ cup Asiago cheese, grated

4 cups cauliflower rice

1 tablespoon lemon juice

1 teaspoon lemon zest

Preparation:

1) Choose the sauté function in the Instant Pot.
2) Add the olive oil and half of the butter.
3) Add the onion.
4) Season with the salt, pepper and red pepper.
5) Cook for 3 minutes.
6) Add the garlic, asparagus and mushroom.
7) Cook for 2 minutes.
8) Add the spinach and peas.
9) Stir until the spinach has wilted.
10) Remove from the pot.
11) Transfer to a large bowl.
12) Stir in the rest of the ingredients before serving.

Serving Suggestion: Garnish with lemon wedges.

Tip: Use freshly squeezed lemon juice.

Nutritional Information Per Serving:

Calories   131

Total Fat 10.4g

Saturated Fat 5.7g

Cholesterol 25mg

Sodium 159mg

Total Carbohydrate 4.9g

Dietary Fiber 1.7g

Total Sugars 2g

Protein 6.2g

Potassium 238mg

89. ARTICHOKE & PEA PASTA

Serves: 2
Preparation time: 1 hour and 15 minutes
Ingredients:

2 tablespoons lemon juice
1 tablespoon lemon zest
2 artichoke hearts
Salt and pepper to taste
4 tablespoons olive oil

2 cloves garlic, crushed and minced
1 cup green peas
¼ cup vegetable broth
3 tablespoons Parmesan cheese, grated
2 cups low carb pasta, cooked

Preparation:

1) Fill a bowl with water. Add the lemon juice.
2) Snap off the outer leaves of the artichokes. Trim the bottom of the stem.
3) Soak the remaining artichokes in the bowl for 30 minutes.
4) Transfer the artichokes and lemon water into your Instant Pot.
5) Seal the pot. Choose manual mode. Cook at high pressure for 10 minutes.
6) Release the pressure quickly.
7) Take the artichokes and let cool.
8) Remove remaining leaves until you see the choke.
9) Remove the tough and feathery parts.
10) Chop the remaining parts.
11) Set the Instant Pot to sauté.
12) Add the oil and sauté the garlic.
13) Add the broth and peas.
14) Simmer for 2 minutes.
15) Add the artichokes and the rest of the ingredients. Mix well.

Serving Suggestion: Sprinkle chopped parsley and red pepper flakes on top of the pasta.
Tip: Choose keto friendly low carb pasta of your choice. You can use linguine or spaghetti.
Nutritional Information Per Serving:

Calories   390
Total Fat 28.9g
Saturated Fat 4.3g
Cholesterol 0mg
Sodium 255mg

Total Carbohydrate 29.6g
Dietary Fiber 12.8g
Total Sugars 6.3g
Protein 10.2g
Potassium 843mg

90. Spaghetti Squash with Bacon & Mushroom

Serves: 4
Preparation time: 20 minutes
Ingredients:

2 lb. spaghetti squash, sliced in half and seeded

4 tablespoons olive oil

3 oz. bacon, chopped

8 oz. mushrooms, sliced

3 cloves garlic, minced

Salt and pepper

¼ cup Parmesan cheese, grated

Preparation:

1) Place the spaghetti squash on top of a steamer rack inside the Instant Pot.
2) Cover the pot.
3) Pour in 1 cup of water.
4) Cook at high pressure for 8 minutes.
5) Do a quick pressure release.
6) Transfer the squash to a plate.
7) Shred using a fork.
8) Press the sauté function in the Instant Pot.
9) Add the oil and bacon.
10) Cook until golden crispy.
11) Add the garlic and mushrooms, and cook for 5 minutes.
12) Season with the salt and pepper.
13) Mix the spaghetti squash with the bacon mixture.

Serving Suggestion: Garnish with fresh sage leaves.

Tip: You can also use ham or sausage in place of bacon.

Nutritional Information Per Serving:

Calories   223
Total Fat 24.4g
Saturated Fat 9.2g
Cholesterol 16mg
Sodium 370mg
Total Carbohydrate 8.5g
Dietary Fiber 0.6g
Total Sugars 1g
Protein 8.6g
Potassium 515mg

Chapter 16: 10 Keto Diet Side Dishes & Desserts

91. Bacon Cheeseburger Dip

Serves: 4
Preparation time: 15 minutes
Ingredients:

6 slices bacon, sliced into small pieces

½ lb. ground beef

10 oz. canned diced tomatoes and green chili peppers

8 oz. cream cheese, cubed

4 tablespoons water

8 oz. cheddar cheese, shredded

Preparation:

1) Set the Instant Pot to sauté.
2) Add the bacon.
3) Cook until golden and crisp.
4) Transfer to a plate lined with paper towel.
5) Add the ground beef, cooked bacon, diced tomatoes, cream cheese and water.
6) Do not stir.
7) Cover the pot.
8) Set it to manual.
9) Cook at high pressure for 4 minutes.
10) Do a quick pressure release.
11) Stir in the cheddar cheese until well combined.

Serving Suggestion: Serve with bell pepper trips or low carb tortilla chips.

Tip: You can skip the green chilli and simply opt for canned tomatoes.

Nutritional Information Per Serving:

Calories   702

Total Fat 54.2g

Saturated Fat 29.7g

Cholesterol 204mg

Sodium 1220mg

Total Carbohydrate 6.2g

Dietary Fiber 1.1g

Total Sugars 2.8g

Protein 47g

Potassium 726mg

92. Creamy Broccoli Mash

Serves: 4
Preparation time: 10 minutes
Ingredients:

1 tablespoon butter
3 cloves garlic, crushed
1 lb. broccoli, chopped
4 oz. cream cheese
½ cup water
Salt and pepper to taste

Preparation:

1) Set the Instant Pot to sauté.
2) Add the butter.
3) Cook the garlic for 30 seconds.
4) Add the rest of the ingredients.
5) Cover the pot.
6) Choose manual mode.
7) Cook at high pressure for 1 minute.
8) Release a pressure quickly.
9) Mash the broccoli.

Serving Suggestion: Sprinkle top with chopped chives.

Tip: Add ¼ teaspoon red pepper flakes if you want the broccoli mash a little spicy.

Nutritional Information Per Serving:

Calories   166
Total Fat 16.2g
Saturated Fat 8.1g
Cholesterol 39mg
Sodium 143mg
Total Carbohydrate 7g
Dietary Fiber 3g
Total Sugars 2g
Protein 5.5g
Potassium 403mg

93. Cauliflower Salad

Serves: 4
Preparation time: 15 minutes
Ingredients:

1 head cauliflower, sliced into florets
4 eggs, hard boiled
1 cup mayonnaise
1 cup bacon bits
2 tablespoons apple cider vinegar
¼ cup onion, chopped
1 teaspoon garlic, minced
¾ cup green onions, chopped
Salt and pepper to taste

Preparation:

1) Place a steamer rack inside the Instant Pot.
2) Add the cauliflower florets on top of the rack.
3) Pour in 1 ½ cups of water.
4) Seal the pot.
5) Set it to manual.
6) Cook at high pressure for 3 minutes.
7) Release the pressure quickly.
8) Remove the cauliflower from the pot.
9) Mash the cauliflower and eggs.
10) Stir in the rest of the ingredients.

Serving Suggestion: Set aside 1 hard-boiled egg, slice into wedges and use these to garnish the salad.

Tip: Use a potato masher to mash the cauliflower.

Nutritional Information Per Serving:

Calories   474
Total Fat 36g
Saturated Fat 8.2g
Cholesterol 210mg
Sodium 1161mg
Total Carbohydrate 10.7g
Dietary Fiber 2.3g
Total Sugars 6.5g
Protein 18.4g
Potassium 497mg

94. DEVILED EGG SALAD

Serves: 4
Preparation time: 25 minutes
Ingredients:

1 tablespoon olive oil

10 eggs

5 strips bacon

2 tablespoons mayonnaise

1 teaspoon Dijon mustard

¼ teaspoon smoked paprika

Preparation:

1) Grease a small cake pan with the olive oil.
2) Crack the eggs into the pan.
3) Pour 1 cup of water into the Instant Pot.
4) Place a steamer rack inside the pot.
5) Put the cake pan on top of the rack.
6) Cover the pot.
7) Choose manual setting.
8) Cook at high pressure for 6 minutes.
9) Release the pressure naturally.
10) Flip the pan onto a chopping board.
11) Chop up the egg.
12) Remove the rack and water from the pot.
13) Set it to sauté.
14) Cook the bacon until golden crisp.
15) Transfer the bacon to a chopping board and chop.
16) Mix the eggs, bacon and the rest of the ingredients.

Serving Suggestion: Garnish with chopped green onion.

Tip: Chill in the refrigerator before serving.

Nutritional Information Per Serving:

Calories   346

Total Fat 26.9g

Saturated Fat 7.5g

Cholesterol 437mg

Sodium 769mg

Total Carbohydrate 3.1g

Dietary Fiber 0.1g

Total Sugars 1.3g

Protein 22.8g

Potassium 287mg

95. BALSAMIC MUSHROOMS

Serves: 4
Preparation time: 15 minutes
Ingredients:
¼ cup olive oil
3 cloves garlic, minced
1 lb. fresh mushrooms, sliced
3 tablespoons balsamic vinegar
Salt and pepper to taste
Preparation:
1) Press the sauté button in the Instant Pot.
2) Add the olive oil.
3) Add the garlic cloves and mushrooms.
4) Toss to coat with oil.
5) Cook for 3 minutes.
6) Add the vinegar.
7) Cook for 2 minutes.
8) Season with the salt and pepper.

Serving Suggestion: Sprinkle top with chopped garlic chives.

Tip: You can also add 3 tablespoons white wine after adding the vinegar.
Nutritional Information Per Serving:
Calories   138
Total Fat 12.9g
Saturated Fat 1.8g
Cholesterol 0mg
Sodium 7mg
Total Carbohydrate 4.6g
Dietary Fiber 1.2g
Total Sugars 2g
Protein 3.7g
Potassium 378mg

96. STRAWBERRY CUPCAKE

Serves: 2
Preparation time: 60 minutes
Ingredients:

½ teaspoon coconut oil

2 eggs

1/3 cup almond flour

2 tablespoons almond milk

½ teaspoon almond extract

¾ teaspoon baking powder

10 drops liquid stevia

2 tablespoons butter, melted

2 strawberries, chopped

Frosting:

2 oz. cream cheese

2 tablespoons butter

1 teaspoon monk fruit sweetener

Liquid stevia to taste

3 teaspoons almond milk

Preparation:

1) Grease 2 muffin cups with coconut oil.
2) In a bowl, beat the eggs.
3) Stir in the almond flour, almond milk, baking powder, stevia, and butter.
4) Pour the batter into the muffin cups.
5) Top with the chopped strawberries. (Set aside some for garnish).
6) Cover with foil.
7) Add a steamer rack inside the Instant Pot.
8) Pour in 2 cups of water. Secure the pot. Choose manual mode.
9) Cook at high pressure for 25 minutes.
10) Release the pressure naturally.
11) Let cool for 15 minutes.
12) In a bowl, mix the cream cheese and butter for 20 seconds using an electric mixer.
13) Add the sweeteners and almond milk, and mix until fluffy.
14) Spread frosting on top of the cupcakes.

Serving Suggestion: Top with the remaining chopped strawberries.

Tip: Do not use monk fruit sweetener with maltodextrin.

Nutritional Information Per Serving:

Calories   455

Total Fat 30.5g

Saturated Fat 19g

Cholesterol 225mg

Sodium 350mg

Total Carbohydrate 4.5g

Dietary Fiber 0.6g

Total Sugars 1.6g

Protein 8.2g

Potassium 155mg

97. Lemon Ricotta Cheesecake

Serves: 6
Preparation time: 60 minutes
Ingredients:

1 teaspoon butter
8 oz. cream cheese
¼ cup and 1 teaspoon Swerve
1 tablespoon lemon juice
1 teaspoon lemon zest
¼ cup ricotta cheese
½ teaspoon lemon extract
2 eggs
2 tablespoons sour cream

Preparation:

1) Coat a small baking pan with butter.
2) In a bowl, mix the cream cheese, ¼ cup Swerve, lemon juice and zest, ricotta cheese and lemon extract.
3) Beat in the eggs.
4) Pour the mixture into the baking pan.
5) Cover with foil.
6) Pour in 2 cups of water into the Instant Pot.
7) Place a steamer rack inside.
8) Put the pan on top of the rack.
9) Seal the pot.
10) Choose manual setting.
11) Cook at high pressure for 30 minutes.
12) Release the pressure naturally.
13) In a bowl, mix the sour cream and remaining Swerve.
14) Spread on top of the cake.

Serving Suggestion: Chill for 6 hours before serving.

Tip: Do not over beat the eggs.

Nutritional Information Per Serving:

Calories   275
Total Fat 25.4g
Saturated Fat 15.3g
Cholesterol 154mg
Sodium 229mg
Total Carbohydrate 3g
Dietary Fiber 0.1g
Total Sugars 0.5g
Protein 9.1g
Potassium 132mg

98. CHOCOLATE CHEESECAKE

Serves: 8
Preparation time: 45 minutes
Ingredients:
Crust:

¼ cup coconut flour

¼ cup almond flour

2 ½ tablespoons cocoa powder (unsweetened)

1 ½ tablespoons low carb sweetener

2 tablespoons butter, melted

Filling:

16 oz. cream cheese

1/3 cup cocoa powder (unsweetened)

½ teaspoon monk fruit powder

2 large egg yolks

1 egg

½ teaspoon stevia powder

1 teaspoon vanilla extract

¾ cup heavy cream

¼ cup sour cream

6 oz. baking chocolate, melted

Preparation:

1) Line a small baking pan with parchment paper.
2) In a bowl, combine all the dry ingredients for the crust.
3) Stir in the butter.
4) Press the mixture into the baking pan.
5) Blend the filling ingredients using a food processor.
6) Pour mixture on top of the crust.
7) Spread it using a spatula.
8) Cover loosely with foil.
9) Place a steamer rack inside the Instant Pot.
10) Put the baking pan on top of the rack.
11) Pour in 1 ½ cups of water. Cover the pot. Set it to manual.
12) Cook at high pressure for 20 minutes.
13) Release the pressure naturally.

Serving Suggestion: Chill in the refrigerator overnight before serving.

Tip: Replace stevia with swerve if not available.

Nutritional Information Per Serving:

Calories 413

Total Fat 38g

Saturated Fat 22g

Cholesterol 153mg

Sodium 56mg

Total Carbohydrates 8g

Dietary Fiber 6g

Sugars 2g

Protein 8g

Potassium 319mg

99. CHOCOLATE MOUSSE

Serves: 4
Preparation time: 30 minutes
Ingredients:

4 egg yolks

¼ cup water

¼ cup cocoa powder (unsweetened)

½ cup Swerve

½ cup almond milk

1 cup whipping cream

½ teaspoon vanilla

¼ teaspoon sea salt

Preparation:

1) In a bowl, beat the egg yolks.
2) Press the sauté function in the Instant Pot.
3) Add the water, cocoa powder and Swerve.
4) Stir until well combined.
5) Add the almond milk and cream.
6) Simmer but do not let it boil.
7) Add the vanilla and salt.
8) Press cancel.
9) Pour the mixture into glass jars.
10) Pour in 1 ½ cups of water into the Instant Pot.
11) Place a steamer rack inside.
12) Put the glass jar on top of the rack.
13) Cover the pot.
14) Choose manual mode.
15) Cook at high pressure for 6 minutes.
16) Do a quick pressure release.

Serving Suggestion: Drizzle top with dark chocolate syrup.

Tip: Refrigerate for 4 hours before serving.

Nutritional Information Per Serving:

Calories   225

Total Fat 21.6g

Saturated Fat 14.2g

Cholesterol 243mg

Sodium 141mg

Total Carbohydrate 6.4g

Dietary Fiber 2.3g

Total Sugars 1.3g

Protein 5g

Potassium 262mg

100. Crème Brulee

Serves: 6
Preparation time: 35 minutes
Ingredients:
6 egg yolks
2 cups heavy whipping cream
5 tablespoons Swerve, divided
1 tablespoon vanilla extract
Preparation:
1) In a bowl, combine the egg yolks, whipping cream, 3 tablespoons sweetener, and vanilla.
2) Mix until well combined.
3) Pour into small ramekins.
4) Cover with foil.
5) Pour 1 cup of water into the Instant Pot.
6) Put a steamer rack inside.
7) Place the ramekins on top of the rack.
8) Cover the pot.
9) Select manual mode.
10) Cook at high pressure for 9 minutes.
11) Let sit for 15 minutes before releasing pressure naturally.
12) Sprinkle remaining sweetener on top.
Serving Suggestion: Refrigerate for 6 hours before serving.
Nutritional Information Per Serving:
Calories   198
Total Fat 19.3g
Saturated Fat 10.8g
Cholesterol 265mg
Sodium 24mg
Total Carbohydrate 2g
Dietary Fiber 0g
Total Sugars 0.4g
Protein 3.5g
Potassium 52mg

Chapter 17: 10 Keto Diet Soups, Broth & Stews

101. Asparagus Soup

Serves: 6
Preparation time: 1 hour and 10 minutes
Ingredients:

3 tablespoons ghee
1 white onion, chopped
5 cloves garlic, crushed
4 cups chicken broth
1 cup ham, diced
2 lb. asparagus, sliced in half
½ teaspoon dried thyme
Salt and pepper to taste

Preparation:

1) Select the sauté function in the Instant Pot.
2) Add the ghee.
3) Add the onion and cook for 5 minutes.
4) Add the garlic, broth and ham.
5) Simmer for 3 minutes.
6) Add the asparagus and thyme.
7) Secure the pot.
8) Choose soup setting.
9) Cook for 45 minutes.
10) Blend the mixture in a food processor.
11) Season with the salt and pepper.

Serving Suggestion: Garnish with low-carb croutons.

Tip: You can also use an immersion blender instead of a food processor.

Nutritional Information Per Serving:

Calories   160
Total Fat 13.4g
Saturated Fat 7.9g
Cholesterol 29mg
Sodium 807mg
Total Carbohydrate 6.9g
Dietary Fiber 4g
Total Sugars 4.1g
Protein 10.7g
Potassium 546mg

102. CHICKEN SOUP

Serves: 4
Preparation time: 30 minutes
Ingredients:

2 tablespoons butter
1 onion, chopped
4 stalks celery, chopped
2 bay leaves
1 carrot, sliced
¼ teaspoon dried oregano

½ teaspoon dried thyme
Salt and pepper to taste
4 cups chicken broth
1 lb. chicken, cooked and shredded
2 cups kale, chopped
½ teaspoon fish sauce

Preparation:

1) Select the sauté function in the Instant Pot.
2) Add the butter.
3) Sauté the onion for 5 minutes.
4) Add the celery, bay leaves and carrot.
5) Season with the oregano, thyme, salt and pepper.
6) Cook for 1 minute.
7) Add the chicken broth.
8) Cover the pot.
9) Set it to manual.
10) Cook at high pressure for 4 minutes.
11) Release the pressure naturally.
12) Add the chicken, kale and fish sauce.
13) Press the sauté button.
14) Simmer for 3 minutes.

Serving Suggestion: Garnish with shredded chicken and chopped green onion.

Tip: You can also use raw chicken, and brown it in the Instant Pot before cooking the onion.

Nutritional Information Per Serving:

Calories   298
Total Fat 16.7g
Saturated Fat 9g
Cholesterol 103mg
Sodium 973mg

Total Carbohydrate 7.2g
Dietary Fiber 1.8g
Total Sugars 2.9g
Protein 39.4g
Potassium 723mg

103. Onion Soup

Serves: 8
Preparation time: 45 minutes
Ingredients:

3 tablespoons avocado oil
8 cups yellow onion, sliced
1 tablespoon balsamic vinegar
6 cups pork stock

2 sprigs fresh thyme
2 bay leaves
1 teaspoon salt

Preparation:

1) Select sauté function in the Instant Pot.
2) Add the avocado oil.
3) Add the onion and cook for 15 minutes, stirring occasionally.
4) Deglaze the pot by pouring in the balsamic vinegar.
5) Scrape the bottom of the pot using wooden spoon.
6) Add the rest of the ingredients.
7) Seal the pot.
8) Choose manual mode.
9) Cook at high pressure for 10 minutes.
10) Release the pressure naturally.
11) Discard the thyme sprigs and bay leaves.
12) Blend the soup using an immersion blender.

Serving Suggestion: Re-heat the soup before serving.

Tip: If you don't have an immersion blender, a regular blender will do.

Nutritional Information Per Serving:

Calories   85
Total Fat 12.8g
Saturated Fat 0.1g
Cholesterol 0mg
Sodium 102mg
Total Carbohydrate 6g
Dietary Fiber 3.7g
Total Sugars 6.5g
Protein 4.8g
Potassium 244mg

104. Beef Pho

Serves: 4
Preparation time: 1 hour and 15 minutes
Ingredients:
Broth:

1 ½ lb. oxtails
5 whole cloves
2 star anise pods
1 cinnamon stick
1/8 teaspoon ground coriander
1 ginger, sliced
½ onion, sliced into quarters

10 cups water
½ lb. beef brisket
Salt to taste
½ Fuji apple, peeled and sliced into chunks
Fish sauce to taste
Swerve or any keto sweetener

Toppings:

6 lb. sirloin steak, sliced
2 zucchinis, spiralized

¼ onion, sliced
2 scallions, sliced and cooked

Preparation:

1) Put the oxtails in a large pot. Cover it with water. Bring to a boil.
2) Turn down the heat. Simmer for 15 minutes.
3) Remove the foam on the surface of the water.
4) Rinse the oxtails. Set aside. Select sauté function in the Instant Pot.
5) Add the cloves, star anise, cinnamon stick and coriander.
6) Toast for 3 minutes, stirring frequently.   Add the ginger and onion.
7) Cook for 2 minutes. Add the water, oxtails, brisket, salt and apple. Cover the pot.
8) Set it to manual. Cook at high pressure for 15 minutes. Release the pressure naturally.
9) Strain the broth. Keep the brisket but discard the onion, apple, spices and ginger.
10) Season with the fish sauce and sweetener.
11) Stir in the zucchini noodles, sirloin steak, onion and scallions.

Serving Suggestion: Garnish with lime wedges and serve with Thai basil and mung bean sprouts.

Tip: You can brown the sirloin steak using the Instant Pot sauté function.

Nutritional Information Per Serving:

Calories   919
Total Fat 34.6g
Saturated Fat 13.3g
Cholesterol 423mg
Sodium 436mg

Total Carbohydrate 5.6g
Dietary Fiber 1.7g
Total Sugars 2.9g
Protein 139g
Potassium 1668mg

105. CARROT SOUP

Serves: 4
Preparation time: 20 minutes
Ingredients:
½ onion, diced
1 clove garlic, minced
8 carrots, sliced into cubes
2 cups vegetable broth
15 oz. coconut milk
Salt and pepper to taste
Preparation:
1) Press the sauté button in the Instant Pot.
2) Add the oil.
3) Sauté onion and garlic for 1-3 minutes.
4) Add the carrots, vegetable broth and coconut milk.
5) Season with the salt and pepper.
6) Seal the pot.
7) Choose manual mode.
8) Cook at high pressure for 8 minutes.
9) Release the pressure naturally.
10) Use an immersion blender to blend the soup until smooth.

Serving Suggestion: Serve this soup with coconut cream and top with chopped parsley.
Tip: You can also use a regular blender to blend the soup.
Nutritional Information Per Serving:
Calories   320
Total Fat 26g
Saturated Fat 22.7g
Cholesterol 0mg
Sodium 482mg
Total Carbohydrate 19.9g
Dietary Fiber 5.7g
Total Sugars 10.5g
Protein 6.1g
Potassium 796mg

106. Taco Soup

Serves: 8
Preparation time: 30 minutes
Ingredients:

1 tablespoon olive oil
2 lb. ground beef
4 cloves garlic, minced
1 tablespoon onion flakes
20 oz. canned diced tomatoes
32 oz. beef broth

2 teaspoons cumin
2 tablespoons chili powder
Salt and pepper to taste
½ cup heavy cream
8 oz. cream cheese

Preparation:

1) Set the Instant Pot to sauté.
2) Pour in the olive oil.
3) Cook the ground beef until brown.
4) Drain excess grease.
5) Add the garlic, onion flakes, diced tomatoes and beef broth.
6) Season with the cumin, chili powder, salt and pepper.
7) Cover the pot.
8) Choose soup setting.
9) Cook for 5 minutes.
10) Release the pressure naturally.
11) Stir in the cream and cream cheese.

Serving Suggestion: Top the soup with sour cream, shredded cheddar cheese and black olives.

Tip: Do not add cream and cream cheese before pressure cooking.

Nutritional Information Per Serving:

Calories 386
Total Fat 28g
Saturated Fat 14g 7
Cholesterol 123mg
Sodium 831mg
Dietary Fiber 1g
Sugars 4g
Total Carbohydrates 8g
Protein 27g
Potassium 261mg

107. CHICKEN BACON CHOWDER

Serves: 4-6
Preparation time: 30 minutes
Ingredients:

6 chicken thighs (boneless), sliced into cubes

½ cup onion, chopped

4 teaspoons garlic, minced

6 oz. mushrooms, sliced

½ cup celery, chopped

8 oz. cream cheese

4 tablespoons butter

Salt and pepper to taste

1 teaspoon thyme

3 cups chicken broth

1 cup heavy cream

2 cups fresh spinach

1 lb. cooked crispy bacon, chopped

Preparation:

1) Place the chicken cubes in a large re-sealable bag.
2) Add the onion, garlic, mushrooms, celery, cream cheese, butter, salt, pepper and thyme.
3) Shake to coat evenly.
4) Store overnight in the refrigerator.
5) The next day, pour the mixture into the Instant Pot.
6) Pour in the chicken broth.
7) Cover the pot.
8) Set it to soup setting.
9) Cook for 30 minutes.
10) Release the pressure naturally.
11) Stir in the cream and spinach.
12) Cover the pot. Let sit for 10 minutes.
13) Sprinkle the bacon bits on top.

Serving Suggestion: Garnish with fresh parsley or fresh herb sprigs.

Tip: The soup pack can be stored in the refrigerator for up to 3 days.

Nutritional Information Per Serving:

Calories   305

Total Fat 29.1g

Saturated Fat 18g

Cholesterol 89mg

Sodium 573mg

Total Carbohydrate 5.2g

Dietary Fiber 1g

Total Sugars 1.5g

Protein 7.3g

Potassium 356mg

108. Buffalo Chicken Soup

Serves: 6
Preparation time: 30 minutes
Ingredients:

1 tablespoon olive oil
1 onion, diced
4 cloves garlic, minced
½ cup celery, diced
1 lb. chicken, cooked and shredded

3 tablespoons Buffalo sauce
4 cups chicken broth
6 oz. cream cheese
½ cup heavy cream

Preparation:

1) Choose the sauté setting in the Instant Pot.
2) Add the oil.
3) Sauté the onion, garlic and celery for 7 minutes.
4) Add the chicken, buffalo sauce and broth.
5) Seal the pot.
6) Select soup mode.
7) Cook for 5 minutes.
8) Release the pressure naturally.
9) Stir in the cream and cheese.
10) Puree in the blender until smooth.

Serving Suggestion: Sprinkle chopped parsley on top.

Tip: Use sugar-free Buffalo sauce.

Nutritional Information Per Serving:

Calories   306
Total Fat 19.2g
Saturated Fat 9.8g
Cholesterol 103mg
Sodium 732mg
Total Carbohydrate 4.4g
Dietary Fiber 0.6g
Total Sugars 1.4g
Protein 27.9g
Potassium 377mg

109. CAULIFLOWER SOUP

Serves: 6
Preparation time: 40 minutes
Ingredients:

6 strips bacon, chopped

¼ cup onion, chopped

2 cloves garlic, minced

1 stalk celery, chopped

Salt and pepper to taste

3 cups chicken broth

1 head cauliflower, sliced into florets

¾ cup sour cream

1 ½ cups cheddar cheese, shredded

Preparation:

1) Turn the Instant Pot to sauté.
2) Add the bacon and cook until golden crisp.
3) Drain on paper towel. Set aside.
4) Cook the onion, garlic and celery in bacon fat for 4 minutes.
5) Season with the salt and pepper.
6) Deglaze the pot by pouring in the chicken broth.
7) Add the cauliflower.
8) Seal the pot.
9) Choose manual setting.
10) Cook at high pressure for 5 minutes.
11) Release the pressure naturally.
12) Stir in the sour cream and cheese.
13) Blend using food processor or immersion blender.
14) Top with the bacon bits before serving.

Serving Suggestion: Serve with low carb toasted bread.

Tip: Celery is optional, and may be replaced by fresh basil.

Nutritional Information Per Serving:

Calories   313

Total Fat 24.1g

Saturated Fat 12.5g

Cholesterol 63mg

Sodium 1027mg

Total Carbohydrate 5.7g

Dietary Fiber 1.4g

Total Sugars 1.9g

Protein 18.5g

Potassium 439mg

110. CABBAGE SOUP

Serves: 10
Preparation time: 20 minutes
Ingredients:

1 tablespoon olive oil
2 lb. ground beef
1 onion, diced
2 cloves garlic, minced
10 oz. canned diced tomatoes with green chili

4 cubes vegetable bouillon, dissolved in ¼ cup water
1 head cabbage, chopped
1 teaspoon ground cumin
Salt and pepper to taste
3 ¾ cups water

Preparation:

1) Choose sauté setting in the Instant Pot.
2) Add the olive oil.
3) Brown the ground beef.
4) Add the onion and garlic.
5) Sauté for 2-3 minutes.
6) Stir in the rest of the ingredients.
7) Cover the pot.
8) Set it to manual.
9) Cook at high pressure for 3 minutes.
10) Release the pressure quickly.

Serving Suggestion: Garnish with the cubed carrot or toasted garlic bits.

Tip: You can add more vegetables such as broccoli or cauliflower if you like.

Nutritional Information Per Serving:

Calories   209
Total Fat 15.2g
Saturated Fat 9.4g
Cholesterol 81mg
Sodium 190mg
Total Carbohydrate 3.5g
Dietary Fiber 2.1g
Total Sugars 2.8g
Protein 28.8g
Potassium 540mg

Chapter 18: 5 Keto Diet Smoothies & Drinks Recipes

111. Mango Ginger Drink

Serves: 4
Preparation time: 10 minutes
Ingredients:
¼ cup mango, chopped
2 tablespoons ginger, minced
4 cups water
Preparation:
1) Place a steamer basket inside the Instant Pot.
2) Add the mango and ginger on top of the basket.
3) Pour in 4 cups of water.
4) Cover the pot.
5) Choose manual mode.
6) Cook at high pressure for 5 minutes.
7) Release the pressure quickly.
8) Chill the water in the refrigerator before drinking.
Serving Suggestion: Garnish with fresh mango cubes.
Tip: Add more water if the flavor is too strong for you.
Nutritional Information Per Serving:
Calories   34
Total Fat 3.3g
Saturated Fat 0.1g
Cholesterol 0mg
Sodium 1mg
Total Carbohydrate 1.1g
Dietary Fiber 1g
Total Sugars 3.7g
Protein 0.6g
Potassium 106mg

112. Raspberry Iced Tea

Serves: 4
Preparation time: 10 minutes
Ingredients:
4 cups water
½ teaspoon baking soda
4 raspberry tea bags
½ cup Swerve
Preparation:
1) Add the water, baking soda and tea bags inside the Instant Pot.
2) Cover the pot.
3) Set it to manual.
4) Cook at high pressure for 4 minutes.
5) Release the pressure naturally.
6) Remove the tea bags.
7) Stir in the sweetener.
8) Chill in the refrigerator before serving.

Serving Suggestion: Sprinkle top with 1 cup chopped fresh raspberry.

Tip: You can also use other keto-friendly sweeteners for this recipe.

Nutritional Information Per Serving:
Calories   64
Total Fat 2.1g
Saturated Fat 0g
Cholesterol 0mg
Sodium 159mg
Total Carbohydrate 2.9g
Dietary Fiber 2.8g
Total Sugars 21.1g
Protein 0.4g
Potassium 76mg

113. Strawberry Milkshake

Serves: 2
Preparation time: 10 minutes
Ingredients:
¼ cup water
¼ cup strawberries, sliced in half
1 cup almond milk (unsweetened)
1 cup crushed ice
¼ cup heavy whipping cream
2 tablespoons Swerve
1 tablespoon cream cheese
½ teaspoon vanilla extract

Preparation:
1) Press sauté setting in the Instant Pot.
2) Add the water.
3) Let it boil.
4) Add the strawberries.
5) Simmer for 5 minutes.
6) Remove the pot.
7) Add the raspberries and the rest of the ingredients in a blender.
8) Blend until smooth.
9) Chill in the refrigerator before serving.

Serving Suggestion: Garnish with the fresh strawberries.
Nutritional Information Per Serving:
Calories 150
Total Fat 15g
Saturated Fat 8g
Cholesterol 41mg
Sodium 250mg
Total Carbohydrates 3.5g
Dietary Fiber 1.5g
Total Sugars 1.5g
Protein 2g
Potassium 50mg

114. Turmeric Coconut Milk

Serves: 4
Preparation time: 40 minutes
Ingredients:

13 oz. coconut milk

3 cups water

2 teaspoons turmeric powder

3 cloves

2 cinnamon sticks

½ teaspoon ginger powder

2 tablespoons Swerve

Preparation:

1) Put all the ingredients except Swerve in the Instant Pot.
2) Mix well.
3) Cover the pot
4) Set it to manual.
5) Cook at high pressure for 15 minutes.
6) Let sit for 10 minutes before release the pressure naturally.
7) Discard the cloves and cinnamon stick.
8) Stir in the sweetener before serving.

Serving Suggestion: Sprinkle top with cinnamon powder.

Tip: This can be served either hot or cold.

Nutritional Information Per Serving:

Calories   110

Total Fat 11.1g

Saturated Fat 9.8g

Cholesterol 0mg

Sodium 10mg

Total Carbohydrate 3.5g

Dietary Fiber 1.5g

Total Sugars 1.6g

Protein 1.1g

Potassium 140mg

115. Peppermint Vanilla Latte

Serves: 6
Preparation time: 20 minutes
Ingredients:
4 cups almond milk
1 teaspoon vanilla
2 cups coffee
3 drops peppermint essential oil
¼ cup Swerve
Preparation:
1) Add all the ingredients in the Instant Pot.
2) Mix well.
3) Cover the pot.
4) Set it to manual.
5) Cook at high pressure for 5 minutes.
6) Release the pressure naturally.
Serving Suggestion: Garnish with fresh peppermint leaves.
Nutritional Information Per Serving:
Calories   278
Total Fat 28.6g
Saturated Fat 25.4g
Cholesterol 0mg
Sodium 19mg
Total Carbohydrate 13g
Dietary Fiber 2.6g
Total Sugars 10.3g
Protein 2.8g
Potassium 345mg

CHAPTER 19: 5 KETO DIET WEEKEND & FESTIVAL RECIPES

116. CHICKEN FAJITAS

Serves: 8
Preparation time: 20 minutes
Ingredients:

4 chicken breasts

Salt and pepper to taste

1 tablespoon fajita seasoning

1 onion, sliced into quarters

2 cloves garlic

1 ½ cup chicken broth

1 teaspoon olive oil

8 low carb tortillas

2 red bell peppers, sliced into strips and grilled

Preparation:
1) Season the chicken breasts with salt, pepper and fajita seasoning.
2) Place inside the Instant Pot.
3) Add the onion and garlic on top of the chicken.
4) Pour in the chicken broth.
5) Lock the lid in place.
6) Set it to manual.
7) Cook at high pressure for 5 minutes.
8) Release the pressure naturally.
9) Let the chicken cool and then shred using a fork.
10) Top the tortillas with shredded chicken and grilled bell peppers and wrap.

Serving Suggestion: You can also add other toppings such as salsa, sour cream, Romaine lettuce, and cilantro.

Tip: You can also sauté the bell pepper in the Instant Pot if you don't have time to grill.

Nutritional Information Per Serving:

Calories   338

Total Fat 12.3g

Saturated Fat 3g

Cholesterol 125mg

Sodium 441mg

Total Carbohydrate 6.8g

Dietary Fiber 4.2g

Total Sugars 2.2g

Protein 43.4g

Potassium 458mg

117. Beef Nachos

Serves: 6
Preparation time: 20 minutes
Ingredients:
1 tablespoon olive oil
2 ½ cups ground beef
1 tablespoon taco seasoning
12 oz. low carb tortilla chips
2 cups cheddar cheese, shredded
3 tablespoons sour cream
Preparation:
1) Set the Instant Pot to sauté.
2) Add the olive oil.
3) Add the ground beef.
4) Season with the taco seasoning.
5) Cook until brown.
6) Arrange the tortilla chips on a baking pan.
7) Spread sour cream on top.
8) Sprinkle cooked beef and cheese.
9) Bake in the oven until the cheese has melted.

Serving Suggestion: Serve with fresh cilantro and salsa.

Tip: You can also use other types of cheese depending on your preference.

Nutritional Information Per Serving:
Calories 778
Total Fat 47g
Saturated Fat 7g
Cholesterol 32mg
Sodium 477mg
Total Carbohydrates 8g
Dietary Fiber 3g
Sugars 1g
Protein 33g
Potassium 158mg

118. Creamy Spicy Deviled Eggs

Serves: 12
Preparation time: 30 minutes
Ingredients:

8 eggs
1 cup cold water
2 tablespoons mayonnaise
1 tablespoon olive oil

1 teaspoon white vinegar
1 teaspoon Dijon mustard
Salt and pepper to taste
½ teaspoon hot sauce

Preparation:

1) Pour the water into the Instant Pot.
2) Place a steamer basket inside.
3) Add the eggs on top of the basket.
4) Close the pot.
5) Choose manual mode.
6) Cook at low pressure for 12 minutes.
7) Release the pressure quickly.
8) Soak the eggs in a bowl with cool water.
9) Peel the eggs.
10) Slice in half and scoop out the yolk.
11) Mash the yolks in a bowl.
12) Add mayonnaise, olive oil, vinegar, mustard, salt, pepper and hot sauce in the bowl.
13) Mix well.
14) Scoop the mixture into the egg whites.

Serving Suggestion: Sprinkle top with paprika.

Tip: You can chill in the refrigerator for a few minutes before serving.

Nutritional Information Per Serving:

Calories   74
Total Fat 15.9g
Saturated Fat 1.4g
Cholesterol 132mg
Sodium 83mg
Total Carbohydrate 1g
Dietary Fiber 0g
Total Sugars 0.5g
Protein 4.5g
Potassium 49mg

119. Barbecue Sliders

Serves: 12
Preparation time: 15 minutes
Ingredients:
4 cups pork strips
1 cup water
2 cups keto-friendly barbecue sauce
12 keto slider buns
Preparation:
1) Season the pork strips with salt and pepper.
2) Place inside the Instant Pot.
3) Pour in the water.
4) Secure the pot.
5) Press the manual button.
6) Cook at high pressure for 10 minutes.
7) Release the pressure naturally.
8) Discard the water.
9) Press the sauté setting.
10) Add the barbecue sauce and simmer for 5 minutes.
11) Put the pork strips inside the Instant Pot.
12) Stuff the slider buns with barbecue meat.

Serving Suggestion: Add Romaine lettuce or avocado cubes to the slider.
Tip: Keto slider buns are made with almond flour.
Nutritional Information Per Serving:
Calories   427
Total Fat 14.5g
Saturated Fat 3g
Cholesterol 24mg
Sodium 1244mg
Total Carbohydrate 31.4g
Dietary Fiber 0.3g
Total Sugars 10.9g
Protein 2.9g
Potassium 132mg

120. Bacon Wrapped Stuffed Chicken Rolls

Serves: 2

Preparation time: 45 minutes

Ingredients:

2 chicken breasts fillets

1 ham, sliced in half

6 asparagus spears, trimmed

8 strips bacon

4 slices Mozzarella cheese

Salt and pepper to taste

Preparation:

1) Flatten the chicken breast using a rolling pin or meat mallet.
2) Season both sides of the chicken fillets with salt and pepper.
3) Place cheese slices, cooked ham and asparagus spears on top of the chicken fillets.
4) Roll each of the fillets tightly.
5) Wrap each chicken roll with bacon slices.
6) Secure with toothpicks.
7) Add 1 cup of water into the Instant Pot.
8) Place a steamer rack inside.
9) Put the chicken rolls on top of the rack.
10) Cover the pot.
11) Choose manual setting.
12) Cook at high pressure for 7 minutes.
13) Release the pressure naturally.
14) Discard the water and remove the rack.
15) Press the sauté setting in the Instant Pot.
16) Cook the rolls until the bacon has turned golden crispy.

Serving Suggestion: Serve with leafy green salad.

Tip: Let cool a little before slicing.

Nutritional Information Per Serving:

Calories   586

Total Fat 41.8g

Saturated Fat 16.5g

Cholesterol 114mg

Sodium 2097mg

Total Carbohydrate 5.9g

Dietary Fiber 1.5g

Total Sugars 1.4g

Protein 45.7g

Potassium 575mg

CONCLUSION

There are many good reasons the ketogenic diet is widely used today in many parts of the world.

As science has proven (and users can attest), it is a highly effective means of losing weight safely. It helps the body burn more fat using the process of ketosis, which was explained in detail in this book.

But that's not all. The keto diet has also been shown to have various benefits for the health—lowering blood pressure and cholesterol levels, reducing the risk of many ailments, improving mental health and many more.

When you make use of this diet, you will not only be able to finally achieve the weight and figure you desire, you can also keep yourself in top health and ward off chronic ailments.

Of course, the diet program is not without drawbacks, risks and side effects. All these were also discussed in this book. The good news is, there are solutions to all of these. The simple solutions and strategies will help you breeze through the adjustment period a lot more easily.

Hopefully, with all the information about the ketogenic diet and the use of Instant Pot provided in this book, along with the 120 delicious and simple keto-friendly recipes, we are able to help you get started with this meaningful journey.
Good luck!

APPENDIX I: MEASUREMENT CONVERSION TABLE

Unit	Conversion	Conversion
1 teaspoon	1/3 tablespoon	1/6 ounce
1 tablespoon	3 teaspoons	½ ounce
1/8 cup	2 tablespoons	1 ounce
¼ cup	4 tablespoons	2 ounces
1/3 cup	¼ cup and 4 teaspoons	2 ¾ ounces
½ cup	8 tablespoons	4 ounces
1 cup	½ pint	8 ounces
1 pint	2 cups	16 ounces
1 quart	4 cups	32 ounces
1 liter	1 quart and ¼ cup	4 ¼ cups
1 gallon	4 quarts	16 cups

APPENDIX II: WEBSITES ABOUT KETO LIFE

Ketogenic.com (https://ketogenic.com/)

Ruled Me (https://www.ruled.me/)

Ketogasm (https://ketogasm.com/)

Diet Doctor (https://www.dietdoctor.com/low-carb/keto)

Keto Connect (https://www.ketoconnect.net/)

The Keto - Weekly Digest for the Keto Community (https://sites.google.com/view/theketo)

Living' La Vida Low-Carb (http://livinlavidalowcarb.com/)

The Ketogenic Diet Resource (http://www.ketogenic-diet-resource.com/)

A Guide to Ketosis (http://josepharcita.blogspot.co.uk/2011/03/guide-to-ketosis.html)

Caveman Keto (http://cavemanketo.com/)

Diet Doctor - LCHF for Beginners (http://www.dietdoctor.com/lchf)

Healthy Keto   (http://healthyketo.com/)

Mona Leigh Sims - Food & Health   (http://www.monasims.com/foodie1.htm)

Peter Attia's Eating Academy (http://eatingacademy.com/)

The Keto Diet   (http://www.reddit.com/r/theketodiet/)

APPENDIX III: RECOMMENDED PRODUCTS FOR KETO DIET

- Ayoba-Yo Spicy Biltong (https://amzn.to/2Lc0qzi)
- Performance Nut Butter (https://amzn.to/2LR2CgQ)
- Dang Lightly Salted Coconut Chips (https://amzn.to/2so3Eca)
- Eden Organic Dry Roasted Pumpkin Seeds (https://amzn.to/2LMsvOJ)
- Zenwise Health Keto-Crave Bars (https://amzn.to/2LPrVjw)
- Moon Cheese (https://amzn.to/2JIW6Ag)
- Hunter Gatherer Wild Sprouted Pili Nuts (https://amzn.to/2JodUL9)
- ChocZero Milk Chocolate Almond Keto Bark (https://amzn.to/2LQsPfC)
- Élan Paleo Mix Granola Shot (https://amzn.to/2JoeJUf)

Made in the USA
Lexington, KY
15 August 2018